Aids to Psychiatry

Aids to Psychiatry

H. G. Morgan

MA, MD (Cantab), FRCP, FRCPsych, DPM (Lond)

Norah Cooke Hurle Professor of Mental Health, University of Bristol;
Honorary Consultant Psychiatrist, South Western
Regional Health Authority

AND

M. H. Morgan

MA, MD (Cantab), FRCP

Consultant Clinical Neurophysiologist, South Western Regional
Health Authority; Clinical Lecturer in Medicine,
University of Bristol

THIRD EDITION

CHURCHILL LIVINGSTONE
EDINBURGH LONDON MELBOURNE AND NEW YORK 1989

CHURCHILL LIVINGSTONE
Medical Division of Longman Group UK Limited

Distributed in the United States of America by
Churchill Livingstone Inc., 1560 Broadway, New
York, N.Y. 10036, and by associated companies,
branches and representatives throughout the
world.

First Edition 1979
Second Edition 1984
Third Edition 1989

ISBN 0-443-03928-3

British Library Cataloguing in Publication Data

Morgan, H. G.
Aids to psychiatry. — 3rd ed.
1. Medicine. Psychiatry
I. Title II. Morgan, M. H., *1934–*
616.89

Library of Congress Cataloging in Publication Data

Morgan, H. G. (Howard Gethin)
   Aids to psychiatry/H. G. Morgan and M. H. Morgan. — 3rd ed.
   Includes bibliographies and index.
   1. Psychiatry. I. Morgan, M. H. (Margaret Hilary) II. Title.
   [DNLM: 1. Mental Disorders. WM 100 M846a]
RC454.M675 1989
616.89–dc 19

Produced by Longman Singapore Publishers (Pte) Ltd.
Printed in Singapore

Preface

This book aims to present the essentials of sound examination technique whether in the writing of answers or in the clinical and viva situation. It is not intended as a substitute for wider reading, and regular reference is made to relevant recent review articles. Although the text is detailed and aimed at postgraduate trainees taking the MRCPsych examination, it is written in such a way that the underlying principles are explained throughout, thereby also making it useful to medical undergraduates.

The approach throughout is to emphasise the marshalling of facts with due regard to their priority and relationship to the realities of clinical practice rather than in an encyclopaedic way. Most important of course is the ability to distinguish essential information from that which is less relevant, particularly with regard to clinical features which are invariable or very common in any condition rather than occasional and infrequent.

A systematic approach to clinical psychiatry and important special topics is followed by consideration of certain aspects of neurology and neurophysiology which the trainee is likely to meet in clinical situations and examinations.

In preparing the third edition, the text has not only been updated but also extended. The sections on organic disorders, the 1983 Mental Health Act and forensic psychiatry are more comprehensive; new topics include childhood sexual abuse and psychiatric aspects of the Auto Immune Deficiency Syndrome (AIDS). The final part concerning examination techniques has also been extensively revised, with a Commentary on the new MRCPsych examination; this is meant to be read in parallel with the remainder of the text, dealing as it does with general principles whereby fact and opinion may be marshalled and presented effectively.

Bristol, 1988   H.G.M
                                                                        M.H.M

Contents

Clinical psychiatry

PART ONE

Clinical psychiatry

Psychopathology

MENTAL PHENOMENA

THOUGHT PROCESSES

Disordered form
Deviation from rational, logical, goal directed thinking.

Autistic thinking
Directed by inner fantasies associated with social withdrawal. Less subject to correction by reality than is normal thinking.

Blocking
Sudden cessation in the flow of thought or speech; occurs in schizophrenia.

Schizophrenic thought disorder
Disturbance in association leading to subtle discontinuities in the flow of speech (knight's move, derailment). May lead to neologisms (newly invented words), or incoherence when severe.

Pressure of speech
Voluble and difficult to interrupt. Often related to anxiety.

Flight of ideas
High speed, leaps from one subject to another connected tenuously together, and distractible in response to environmental stimuli. Speech voluble. Often includes punning. Common in hypomanic illness.

Clang associations
Dictated by chance sounds of words rather than their meanings. Often associated with flight of ideas.

Retardation
Slowing of speech as in depression when it may be part of a general picture of psychomotor retardation.

Mutism
Refusal to speak whether for conscious or unconscious reasons.

Disordered content

Obsessional ruminations
The pathological presence of a persistent and repetitive thought, feeling or impulse that cannot be eliminated from consciousness by deliberate effort. On quiet reflection the patient recognises that it has no rational basis and that it is due to his own psychological processes rather than some outside influence. Resistance to it is accompanied by anxiety. In obsessive compulsive neurosis may lead to severe disturbance in behaviour.

Delusions
A belief that is firmly held against all evidence to the contrary and which is out of context with the person's educational and cultural background. It is incorrigible, often centred on the self (egocentric) and usually, but not necessarily, false.

Types
Paranoid: ideas of persecution and injustice.
Depressive: morbid guilt, self blame, futility.
Hypochondriacal: concern with bodily and personal attributes and may be bizarre.
Grandiose: over-estimation of personal qualities, abilities, finances (as in hypomanic illness).
Passivity: abnormal influences on bodily processes by outside agencies (as in schizophrenic illness).
Reference: excessive focus of attention from others, often associated with undue sensitivity or paranoid ideation.
Autochthonous (apophanous): sudden onset, fully elaborated apparently not related to situations or current preoccupation (in schizophrenia).
Secondary: follows some other morbid experience. For example, severe depression with morbid guilt may lead to belief that others will share that view of him and behave towards him accordingly.
Systematised: usually in chronic schizophrenic psychosis, when a rational internal consistency between various delusions is developed.

COGNITIVE FUNCTION

Level of consciousness
Organic states may lead to confusion in which there is disorientation in time, place and person, with feelings of bewilderment. In clouding of consciousness there is similar disturbance of perception and

attention with subsequent amnesia. When there is also marked anxiety a state of delirium exists when there may also be hallucinations, paranoid ideation and consequently overactive or aggressive behaviour.

Coma
Profound loss of consciousness due to organic cause. Deepest levels may be associated with loss of all responses and even reflexes.

Stupor
A state of relative non-responsiveness to the environment. May be part of pre-coma in organic disturbance, electrolyte disorders, mid brain tumours, hypoglycaemia. The psychogenic type (depressive or catatonic or hysterical) associated with full awareness of environment.

Patient is immobile, mute, eyes may follow external object. EEG may be useful in diagnosis.

Attention
In the normal state this involves a central focus of high intensity with extension to include a variable amount of peripheral material in a less clear way. Both intensity and extent of attention may be impaired by psychological and organic factors, often in a fluctuant way.

Variability is a marked feature of early organic impairment.

Distractibility is common in hypomanic euphoria.

Intense preoccupation with a single theme may occur in depression (guilt) or obsessional states (phobic objects or rituals).

Selective inattention is similar to the defence of denial with avoidance of matters that generate anxiety.

In hypnosis there is restricted awareness with intense focus on one area of consciousness and heightened suggestibility.

Orientation
The ability to recognise one's surroundings and their temporal and spatial relationship to oneself, or to appreciate one's relationship to the environment.

This requires adequacy of exteroceptive data, effective recent memory and correct intellectual adjustment to outer reality (level of consciousness, freedom from delusional thinking).

Concerns
Time: (hour, day, week and year).
Place: (present location, its nature, home address, reasons for being in present situation).
Person: (Identity of self and others).

May be related to organic disorder but psychogenic factors may lead to disorientation as in hysterical dissociation.

Memory

Registration
Impaired by any reduction in consciousness and awareness. Alcohol, drug induced or other organic disorders of the central nervous system. Psychogenic factors include severe anxiety and panic states.

Retention
Extremely rapid decay in 'curve of forgetting' may occur in certain organic brain diseases, e.g. Korsakoff's Psychosis. In Alzheimer's disease there is a profound impairment of new learning, but in the early stages the rate of forgetting, once information is acquired, may be normal.

Recall
Amnesia is the partial or total inability to recall past experiences. Psychogenic impairment usually related to emotional difficulties, selective for painful events, either recent or distant, and memories may return. In gross hysterical state there may be global amnesia involving all past events and identity. May be associated with physical flight to new and strange surroundings (fugue). Organic amnesia may be irreversible, usually concerns recent events and may leave remote memory intact and not specifically selective for emotionally traumatic events. Important to note that typical hysterical amnesia may occur in addition to underlying organic brain disorder, and may even be precipitated by it.

Recognition
A sense of familiarity concerning recalled material. In mild nominal dysphasia words may be correctly recognised and identified even though their spontaneous recall is not possible.

Deja vu
Illusion of recognition in which a new situation is incorrectly regarded as a repetition of a previous memory. Common in normal anxiety states or epileptic aura.

Jamais vu
Illusion of failure to recognise familiar situations.

Confabulation
The filling of gaps in memory by false imagined experiences which the patient believes to be true.

Dysphasia and aphasia
Specific memory disorder for words and language related to organic brain disturbance in the dominant temporal lobe (speech centre), and contiguous areas.

Intelligence

Ability to solve problems which require logical thought processes. Considerable normal individual differences in accuracy, speed, level of problem complexity and flexibility as well as originality of solution.

Routine clinical assessment of intelligence permits only approximate estimation. Poor educational experience, sociocultural factors or mental illness must always be allowed for before a judgement is made. Standardised intelligence tests are highly reliable and should always be used when routine clinical assessment suggests that further investigation of intelligence level is needed.

$$\text{Intelligence quotient (I.Q.)} = \frac{\text{mental age (Binet Simon scale)}}{\text{chronological age}} \times 100$$

PERCEPTION

The awareness of objects, qualities and relations that follow stimulation of peripheral sensory organs as distinct from awareness that results from memory.

Illusions

Perceptual misinterpretation of a real external sensory experience. Often dictated by dominant affective state, e.g. anxiety which may lead to threatening distortion of visual experiences.

Hallucinations

Apparent perception of an external object in the absence of an adequate sensory stimulus. An internal psychological event is mistakenly attributed to an external source.

Any sensory modality may be involved: may refer to external surroundings or to bodily function.

When caused by organic factors there may be impaired consciousness. Organic causes include hallucinogenic drugs, epilepsy, delirium due to toxic agents or alcohol/barbiturate withdrawal states. Psychogenic causes include schizophrenic psychosis which typically occurs in the setting of clear consciousness. May be hypnagogic (preceding sleep) or hypnopompic (on waking).

AFFECT

The feeling tone that accompanies ideation. Synonymous with emotion. Mood refers to a sustained affective state. Affect may be shallow, inappropriate (does not relate to stimuli or situation), labile, or qualitatively changed as in depression, euphoria, anxiety or anger. Consequent behaviour changes such as aggression may be closely associated with disorders of affect.

Anxiety
An unpleasant emotional state characterised by feelings of apprehension, impending threat or danger. Associated with characteristic pattern of somatic and autonomic changes such as increased sweating, tremor, dry mouth, tachycardia and subjective feelings of tension. May be either free floating, or phobic when it is focussed on specific objects or situations.

Depression
Varies from mild dejection to deep melancholia and despair. Often closely associated with anxiety. When severe there may be secondary disorders of ideation (self blame and futility, hypochondriasis, suicidal thoughts) and of behaviour (retardation, self neglect or agitation when anxiety is also marked).

Euphoria and elation
Elevation of mood with feelings of emotional and physical well being combined with optimism concerning the life situation. When pathological it is usually quite clearly excessive and inappropriate, and may then be accompanied by over-confidence, increased motor activity and impaired judgement.

Ambivalence
The coexistence of opposite emotions and attitudes towards a given object or situation. A common cause of mood swings or oscillation between mild euphoria and depression/anxiety (cyclothymia).

Depersonalisation
A feeling of unreality and strangeness concerning one's own person. May feel outside the self, observing it objectively and feeling separate from it. May occur in normals especially with fatigue, or in epilepsy, psychosis (depressive or schizophrenic) or as a hysterical phenomenon.

Derealisation
Loss of sense of reality concerning one's surroundings. Closely associated with depersonalisation. May occur together with severe anxiety in certain phobic states.

GENERAL BEHAVIOUR

Closely related to affective, cognitive and perceptual mental function.

Over-activity
Agitation is a state of restless motor activity that is a manifestation of emotional tension.

Hyperkinesis in children may be related to organic or emotional disturbance.

General increase in activity may be related to euphoric mood states.
Focussed on compulsions and rituals in obsessive compulsive states.

Under-activity
Depressive retardation may lead to slowing of response and ultimate stupor. Psychasthenic states due to anxiety may limit activities because of feelings of fatigue and exhaustion.

Catatonic stupor in schizophrenic patients may lead to prolonged periods of inactivity.

Self neglect
May be related to:
— retardation and ideas of futility in depressive psychosis.
— preoccupation with fantasies and delusions in schizophrenia.
— excitement and lack of judgement in hypomania.
— intellectual impairment in dementia.

Abnormal movements
Stereotypies: the frequent repetition of any speech or action.
Common in chronic schizophrenia.
Mannerisms: idiosyncratic elaboration of normal movements, common in chronic schizophrenia.

Compulsions
Occur as part of an obsessional state. Repetitive, stereotyped motor acts, usually secondary to obsessional ideas: e.g. hand washing follows idea of contamination. Only transient reduction of anxiety achieved.

Echolalia
Pathological repetition by imitation of speech of another person.
Called echopraxia when this involves imitation of movement.

Flexibilitas cerea
Maintenance of imposed posture as in hypnosis or catatonic schizophrenia.

Negativism
Resistance to suggestion, tending to do the opposite, as seen in catatonic schizophrenia.

INSIGHT
Full insight requires a correct understanding of the severity, implications and causes of one's illness.

A psychotic patient may not recognise the presence of illness and may fail to accept any such proposition. He may later recover only partial insight, accepting that he had previously been ill but remaining unwilling to agree to its psychiatric nature.

Neurotic illness is characterised by insight into the fact of disability, through true awareness of the nature of the underlying psychological factors is often absent.

The chronic brain syndrome (dementia) may lead to severe loss of insight because of impaired judgement secondary to loss of memory and other intellectual abilities. Acute clouding of consciousness also impairs insight.

FURTHER READING

Kopelman, M. D. (1987) Amnesia: organic and psychogenic. *Brit. J. Psychiat.*, **150**, 428–443.
Lishman, W. A. (1987) *Organic Psychiatry*, 2nd edn. Oxford: Blackwell Scientific.

MENTAL MECHANISMS

Psychoanalytic theory proposes that during development defence strategies are used to mediate between unconscious instinctual drives and the strictures of outside reality.

The repertoire of defences which an individual possesses dictates his character traits.

Defences occur as part of normal development and everyday life: they are not in themselves pathological unless they become excessive or fail to maintain adequate functioning of the individual. Defences may be classified according to the libidinal phase at which they arise, or according to the psychopathology with which they are associated, or whether they are basic or composite.

Repression
Given a central position by Freud. Leads to inability to remember unpleasant wishes or impulses. Common in hysterical, dissociative behaviour but may occur as part of other defences, e.g. sublimation.

Displacement
Shifting of emotion from one idea or object to another in a way that causes less anxiety and guilt.

Reaction formation
An unacceptable impulse is transformed into its opposite. Common in obsessive compulsive neurosis.

Isolation
Separation of an idea from the affect which accompanies it.

Undoing
Attempts to cancel out a previously committed act by counter actions. Characteristic of obsessive compulsive states with

expiatory rituals which attempt to undo some forbidden act or cancel the effects of a wish to which has been attributed imaginary power of action.

Rationalisation
This provides alternative explanation for instinctual motives and drives.

Intellectualisation
Excessive use of intellectual processes to avoid affective experience.

Denial
May refer to the affect associated with an idea or event or may include the whole episode. Exclusion from conscious memory.

Projection
One's own feelings and wishes are attributed to another person. Common in normals and fundamental in paranoid psychosis.

Regression
A return to an earlier state of psychological development in order to avoid tension and conflict of the present. Common in normals under stress as well as in pathological states.

Counterphobic mechanisms
Attempt to alleviate phobic anxieties by excessive activity in specific relation to the area of concern.

Withdrawal and avoidance
Removal of the self from conflict situations. This may lead to a failure to resolve them.

Introjection
Qualities of a loved object are internalised and the distinction between it and the self tends to be minimised or obliterated. This attempts to reduce painful awareness of separateness and loss.

Identification
Usually with a loved object: may also be dictated by guilt.

Acting out
The living out (in action) of warded-off memories when the links between the action and the memory are obscure to the patient.

Sublimation
Psychic energy is deflected to another goal which is more acceptable to the individual concerned.

Problems of terminology and classification

THE WHO INTERNATIONAL CLASSIFICATION OF DISEASES (ICD 9th Revision 1978)

Statistical classification of mental disorders and related conditions. The section concerning mental disorders is the only one which contains a glossary of terms. This reflects special problems posed by lack of independent laboratory information. In the ICD each condition has a 3-digit number code, each with subcategories 0.1–0.9.

THE DIAGNOSTIC AND STATISTICAL MANUAL OF MENTAL DISORDERS (DSMIIIR 1987)

Compiled by the American Psychiatric Association. Uses a multiaxial classification. Emphasises description and it aims to be atheoretical. It has discarded terms such as endogenous/reactive, and neurosis/psychosis. Each condition is categorised along five distinct axes. These are:

Axis I   The Mental Disorders
Axis II   Personality Disorders and Specific Developmental Disorders
Axis III   Associated Physical Disorders
Axis IV   Severity of Psychosocial Stressors
Axis V   Highest Level of Adaptive Functioning in the Past Year

NEUROSIS

PSYCHONEUROSIS

When Freud introduced this term, he used it to refer to a disabling symptom as well as to a process involving unconscious conflict leading to anxiety. This in turn produces maladaptive defence mechanisms which result in symptoms.

NEUROTIC DISORDER

In ICD9 this is characterised by the following criteria:
— no demonstrable organic basis
— considerable insight: unimpaired reality testing, no confusion with morbid subjective experiences or fantasies having external reality
— behaviour may be abnormal, although it usually remains within socially acceptable limits
— personality not disorganised
— principal manifestations include: excessive anxiety, hysterical symptoms, phobias, obsessional and compulsive symptoms, depression.

NEUROTIC PROCESS

DSMIII attempts to exclude theoretical assumptions in defining neurotic disorders, and uses a separate term, 'Neurotic Process', which refers to a specific aetiological mechanism involving unconscious conflict leading to defence mechanisms that result in symptoms and/or personality disturbance.

PSYCHOSIS

Implies major break with reality and impaired insight.
ICD9 distinguishes:
  organic psychosis due to impaired cognitive function
  other psychoses (including the Schizophrenias and Affective Psychoses) characterised by delusions.
The term psychosis is unsatisfactory because:
— it includes a wide variety of disparate conditions
— criteria are not easily measured (e.g. insight, understandability)
— particular problems in Depressive Disorders which are not easily classified as neurotic or psychotic, either from the point of view of description or aetiology
— criteria of severity not always useful (for example, some neurotic disorders may appear to be more disabling than psychotic ones)
— hallucinatory experiences can occur in other conditions (for example, hysterical states).

Organic disorders

A. ENDOCRINE, METABOLIC AND DEFICIENCY DISORDERS

THYROTOXICOSIS

May present with psychological symptoms, which are almost invariably present.

Common. Anxiety, hyperactivity, emotional lability. Often no preceding history of anxiety and may be no psychological precipitants.

Less common. Depression with agitation or apathy, early morning waking. May persist after return to euthyroid state, and require antidepressant therapy. Euphoria or 'hypomanic veneer'.

Rare. Acute organic confusion (in severe toxicity), schizophrenic reaction.

Physical. Weight loss in spite of good appetite, intolerance of hot weather, sleeping pulse more than 90/minute, atrial fibrillation.

HYPOTHYROIDISM (Myxoedema)

Basically an organic mental syndrome with secondary psychological features depending upon personality type. Most common in the elderly. When it occurs in infancy or childhood it may lead to mental handicap if it remains untreated; it is reversible if treated early.

Common. Memory impairment, dulled comprehension. May lead to irreversible dementia. Depression with lethargy, irritability (may present in this way): can persist after return to euthyroid state and require antidepressant therapy.

Less common. Coma: may present in this way, often precipitated by infection, high mortality when hypothermia also present. (< 35°C). Excessive suspiciousness, paranoid and hallucinatory psychosis. Mania.

14

Physical features. Cold sensitivity, physical slowness, weight increase, non-pitting oedema (pretibial), facial puffiness, hoarse voice, coarse dry skin, thinning of hair, carpal tunnel syndrome, angina (secondary to hypercholesterolaemia).

Richard Asher coined the term 'myxoedema madness' to include a wide variety of psychiatric states.

VITAMIN B₁ (thiamine) DEFICIENCY

See Wernicke's encephalopathy (pp. 19, 114) and Korsakoff's psychosis (pp. 25, 114).

VITAMIN B 12 DEFICIENCY

Distinctive. Memory deficits, poor concentration: found in 25% of patients with Addisonian anaemia. May precede neurological and haematological abnormality. Screen for B12 deficiency: all undiagnosed organic brain syndromes, especially in elderly, post-gastrectomy, other intestinal diseases, severe chronic dietary deficiency. May be progressive dementia in severe cases.

Non-specific. Affective disorder (anxiety, irritability, depression) in 20%. Folic acid deficiency is said to be more likely to cause affective disorder (56%).

NICOTINIC ACID DEFICIENCY (Pellagra)

Tryptophan deficient diets. Neglect of diet in elderly. Secondary to chronic diarrhoea. Initial depression. Later confusion, delirium and dementia.

HEPATIC ENCEPHALOPATHY

A range of neuropsychiatric disorders associated with hepatic insufficiency.

Clinical features
Chronic organic brain syndrome punctuated by episodic disorders of consciousness, with or without delirium, and finally coma.

In early stages:
— exaggeration of personality traits
— anxiety, depression or denial
— reversal of sleep rhythm
— slowing of EEG
— fluctuating degrees of concentration, awareness
— constructional apraxia

In later stages:
— confusion, inappropriate behaviour
— delusional ideas, hallucinations
— visual illusions (micropsia)
— hepatic coma (may be heralded by stupor, fits, flapping tremor of hands, hypertonia and hyper-reflexia, extensor plantar responses)

Causes
Due to metabolic changes secondary to liver cell failure. Precise metabolites involved uncertain:
— raised blood ammonia usually found but its level does not correlate closely with severity of symptoms
— toxic products of protein breakdown (such as methionine and tryptophan metabolites) entering systemic blood supply via new collateral extrahepatic and intrahepatic shunts
— short chain fatty acids may also be toxic
— accumulation of neurotransmitters originating from bacterial protein breakdown in gut
— coma may be precipitated by diuretics, high protein intake, presence of blood in gut, intercurrent infection, sedatives, phenothiazines, monoamine oxidase inhibitors and other antidepressants. Portal systemic shunt (especially if surgically induced in treatment of portal hypertension) may be cause of delusional hallucinatory symptoms and central nervous damage (paraplegia, cerebellar and basal ganglion disease, epileptic fits).

Differential diagnosis
Important to distinguish alcoholic delirium tremens from hepatic encephalopathy if only because sedatives can be fatal in latter.

Liver failure	*DTs*
Hypoactive apathetic state	Physically overactive
May resemble depression	Vivid visual hallucinations, severe anxiety
Irregular flapping tremor may occur	Tremor coarse, rhythmic
EEG: progressive slowing with high amplitude triphasic waves	

CUSHING'S DISEASE

Due to excess production of cortisol with variable amount of adrenal androgens. Adenoma or carcinoma of adrenal cortex (20%) adrenal hyperplasia (80%). Psychological symptoms in >50%: more likely when history of previous psychiatric difficulties, improve with adequate treatment of endocrine disorder.

Common. Depression with anxiety or retardation, excessive fatigue, stupor, episodic acute excitement, anxiety, impotence, amenorrhoea, loss of libido. Severity of depression not related to levels of circulating cortisol: it may be rapidly relieved when tumour or hyperplastic gland removed. Tumour less commonly associated with psychiatric symptoms than is hyperplasia.

Less common. Paranoid delusions, auditory hallucinations. Elation, euphoria (2%). Acute organic reactions: may be subjective complaint of memory impairment when objective findings minimal.

ADDISON'S DISEASE

Chronic adrenocortical insufficiency of cortisol, aldosterone, corticosterone and androgens. Primary atrophy (up to 50%). In the past tuberculosis more common. Psychological symptoms present in all severe cases. Mild memory impairment (75%). Organic type symptoms vary with severity of underlying endocrine deficiency and hypoglycaemia: in crisis there may be delirium. Depression (25%), apathy (25%), irritability (up to 50%). Rare to see other psychotic symptoms.

ACTH AND CORTICOSTEROID THERAPY

Psychological symptoms more likely with high doses or prolonged treatment, or history of previous psychiatric difficulties. Euphoria (up to 70%). Depression far less common (contrast Cushing's Disease). Irritability, tension. Psychosis (5%): mania, depression, stupor, disorientation, delusions, hallucinations, catatonia. Psychological dependence, with depression as a result of steroid withdrawal, sometimes occurs.

HYPOPITUITARISM

Chronic anterior pituitary failure. Most commonly due to post-partum ischaemic necrosis. Early loss of libido, pubic and axillary hair. Skin pale, wrinkled. Weight loss not a significant feature. Depression, apathy, self neglect. Sensitivity to cold. Sleepy. Memory impairment. Episodes of confusion, delirium, liability to become comatose and die in absence of endocrine replacement.

PHAEOCHROMOCYTOMA

May lead to episodic symptoms which mimic acute anxiety. Usually severe headache. Often precipitated by emotional arousal or physical exertion.

INSULINOMA

Episodic behaviour which may be out of character, aggression, confusion and loss of consciousness in severe cases.

FURTHER READING

Lishman, W. A. (1978) *Organic Psychiatry*. Oxford: Blackwell.

RENAL ENCEPHALOPATHY

Clinical features
May be due to
— uraemia
— underlying disease process
— secondary physical and psychological complications

Uraemic encephalopathy
Essentially an organic brain syndrome. Psychological disturbance found in 75% of patients who have blood urea of more than 250 mg%. At first: fatigue, headache, poor concentration. Later: episodic confusion or delirium, coma.

Neurological disorder
Myoclonic jerks, asterixis, (metabolic flap) usually at times of clouded consciousness, extrapyramidal rigidity, involuntary movements, neuropathy (painful paraesthesiae, restless legs syndrome), polymyositis (proximal limb weakness), epileptic fits (33%), reversible amaurosis.

EEG changes
Degree of abnormality correlated with level of consciousness. Generalised slow wave activity, disorganisation, episodic semi-rhythmic slow waves, may be triphasic forms, abnormal arousal responses. Spontaneous paroxysmal epileptiform abnormalities, also induced by photic stimulation, with or without convulsions. Poor correlation with blood urea levels; other metabolic changes interact.

Dialysis: marked EEG changes during or after, especially if dialysis disequilibrium syndrome, features as above in uraemia. Chronic dementia of dialysis: diffuse slow waves, superimposed rhythmic high amplitude slow waves, triphasic waves, complex discharges. May precede clinical change, and made transiently worse by dialysis.

Psychological disturbance
Depression: early features of uraemia may mimic this, but may develop secondarily.
Anxiety
Secondary defence mechanisms

Aetiology

Neuropathological. Some neuronal degeneration and loss. May be overshadowed by vascular complications due to secondary disorders such as hypertension. Urea itself not neurotoxic.

Electrolyte and acid/base changes. Especially when these are rapid.

Water intoxication

Abnormal neurotransmitter metabolism

Wernicke's encephalopathy: thiamine deficiency.

Iatrogenic. High doses of penicillin may cause fits. Diuretics may cause hypokalaemia. Immunosuppressants and steroids may predispose to viral or fungal meningoencephalitis or reticulo-endothelial tumours.

Effects of dialysis
When carried out rapidly or there is severe initial metabolic abnormality, then dialysis may lead to a 'disequilibrium syndrome' of headache, confusion, fits, coma. This may be due to cerebral oedema, or reactive hypoglycaemia may also be a factor.
   Dementia may also complicate dialysis. Usually progressive and fatal in few months, often with osteomalacia, multiple bone fractures, orofacial grimacing and fits. Appears to be unrelated to biochemical disturbance, and not improved by further dialysis. May be due to accumulation in brain of aluminium derived from water used in dialysis.

Hospital ward regimes
May involve social isolation and sensory deprivation. These may heighten anxiety, accentuate confusion, precipitate delirium or paranoid reaction.

Renal transplantation donors
Careful psychological screening of potential donors.
Sudden irrational decision suspect especially when family coercion present.

Exclude donor who has markedly ambivalent relationship with recipient.

B. ORGANIC BRAIN SYNDROMES

CHARACTERISTIC CLINICAL FEATURES

Tend to show marked fluctuation in severity, worse at night.
1. Memory loss (most severe for recent events).
2. Impairment of consciousness (especially in acute forms).
3. Disorientation (time, place, person).
4. Intellectual impairment (defect of grasp, reasoning, social disinhibition).
5. Non-specific: hallucinations (especially visual), mood disturbances (lability, depression), delusional ideas, focal neurological signs.

ACUTE ORGANIC BRAIN SYNDROMES

Disorientation and clouding of consciousness predominate. May also be anxiety, bewilderment, illusions, hallucinations (delirium).

Causes
Metabolic, infective, toxic, traumatic, degenerative, vascular. Alcohol or barbiturate withdrawal in habituated individuals, nutritional deficiency. Wernicke's encephalopathy (thiamine deficiency), begins with global confusional state, drowsiness, inattention, disorientation, failure of identification. Nystagmus and ocular palsies frequent, and delirium tremens in a third. Emergency need for treatment with intramuscular thiamine 50 mg daily. Rapid recovery possible, but may only be partial.

CHRONIC ORGANIC BRAIN SYNDROME

The dementias
Dementia is a syndrome arising from cerebral disease, primarily causing impaired recent memory, with additional variable disturbance of intellect, abstract thinking, judgement, personality, affect and higher cortical functions (e.g. orientation, speech). It occurs in the absence of any alteration in consciousness, but may cause episodic confusion or delirium. The loss of intellectual abilities interferes with social or occupational functioning. Progressive selective deficits imply focal dysfunction. 3–5% of people over 65 years have severe dementia, similar proportion milder effect. 80% over 80 years are not demented.

History
Essential to have objective information from relatives, friends and work colleagues to ascertain change from premorbid function, duration, speed of onset and evidence of selective difficulty. Family history in case of inherited disorders, e.g. Huntington's Chorea.

Examination
To assess degree of deficit as well as possible causes.
a) Full general physical for evidence of systemic disease, e.g. metabolic or neoplastic.
b) Neurological for focal cranial nerve or limb signs. N.B. Look for apraxia — a defect of action inexplicable by simple motor or sensory loss — implies parietal lobe involvement.
c) Simple tests of mental function:
   1. Language:
     i) naming objects:
      — nominal dysphasia if single nouns.
      — expressive dysphasia if more extensive disability.
     ii) spoken commands:
      — receptive dysphasia — failure to understand single words or sentences.
      — dyslexia — reading disability. If comprehension and speech intact, indicates dominant hemisphere parieto-occipital lesion.
      — dysgraphia — writing disorder.
   2. Calculation — 7s subtracted serially from 100 (is also a test of concentration).
     — dyscalculia.
   3. Spatial organisation — drawing a star or a cube.
   4. Short term memory — digit span, usually more than 5 forward.
   5. Problem solving — e.g. placing digits in reverse order.
   6. Recent memory — recalling current events. Babcock sentence or 3 unrelated words and a simple address.
d) Where doubt remains and/or suspicion of selective deficits, then detailed psychometric assessment may be required.

Causes, presentation

Cerebral atrophy (50%). Senile dementia; Alzheimer senile (50–70% of patients over 65) and pre-senile types. Early memory loss, dressing apraxia, disorientation, fits, extrapyramidal signs. Neuronal loss, argentophil plaques, neurofibrillary cell changes. Marked involvement of parietal lobes. Pick's disease (rare). Mendelian dominant. Early social disinhibition (frontal lobe involvement). Rigid egocentric attitude. Focal neurological deficits common, e.g. dysphasia. Memory loss late. Neuronal loss, presence of balloon-like Pick cells.

Cerebrovascular disease Multi-infarct dementia (10–30%). Affects thalamus, basal ganglia, brainstem and cerebrum. Can be coincidental with dementia from other causes. Depression often marked initially.

Alcoholic dementia (5–10%). Cortical atrophy in excess of age effect. 5–10%). Cortical atrophy in excess of age effect.

Normal pressure hydrocephalus (Adams syndrome) (6%). Psychomotor retardation, ataxia and urinary incontinence. Insidious onset, ventricular enlargement, normal CSF pressure. May occur after head injury, subarachnoid haemorrhage, intracranial surgery, cerebrovascular disease, meningo-encephalitis, with brainstem glioma, third ventricular cyst, cerebellar tumour, aqueduct stenosis.
   In half there is no obvious cause.
   Important because improvement can follow introduction of intracerebral shunt. Selection and investigation of patients needs care as significant morbidity associated with treatment.

Huntington's chorea (3%). Dominant autosomal inheritance. Incidence 5/100 000. Some sporadic cases occur (mutation). Onset 30–50 years of age. May be depression or paranoid state initially. Increased family incidence of suicide, antisocial behaviour. All children of an affected parent have 50% chance of developing the disease.

Parkinson's disease. This together with normal pressure hydrocephalus and Huntington's chorea sometimes called 'subcortical dementias' (see below).

Chronic drug intoxication (3%).

Miscellaneous diseases (7–10%).
   — Traumatic. Degree of dementia correlates well with duration of post-traumatic amnesia (duration after injury before continuous memory recall is established).
   — Punch-drunk syndrome. Cerebral atrophy, which progresses until retirement from the ring, only occasionally afterwards. Cerebellar, pyramidal, extrapyramidal signs, morbid jealousy, impotence.
   — Metabolic. Hypothyroidism, when chronic and severe. Hypoglycaemia (intermittent disordered behaviour, confusion or loss of consciousness more common than a true dementia). Chronic renal dialysis, related to accumulation of aluminium from dialysis fluid. Hyperadrenalism, Cushing's syndrome. Hepatic failure. Addisonian anaemia.
   — Infective. Neurosyphilis: (general paralysis of the insane; G.P.I; tabo-paresis). May present with depression, grandiose

paranoid psychosis (10%), social disinhibition. Human autoimmune deficiency syndrome (AIDS).
— Hypoxic. Coal gas poisoning: beware late deterioration after 10 days.
— Other neurological disorders. There may be inappropriate euphoria in multiple sclerosis; frontal lobe tumours can cause disinhibited behaviour. Dementia with Parkinson's disease, with cerebellar atrophy e.g. Ramsay-Hunt syndrome, neurosyphilis, Creutzfeldt-Jakob disease, chronic undetected subdural haematoma.

'Subcortical dementias'

Impaired cerebral function can arise from subcortical lesions in several sites, but the clinical presentations tend to be similar — personality change, impaired memory, particularly retrieval, impaired information processing and ability to manipulate acquired knowledge. May appear depressed, but in reality lack initiative, are slow but antidepressants cause further cognitive difficulty. The functions of language, calculation, and learning remain intact — unlike the cortical dementias.

Pathology affects subcortical grey or white matter or both.

Causes include some frontal lobe tumours, the deterioration associated with progressive supra-nuclear palsy, Huntington's chorea, Parkinson's disease and other extra-pyramidal syndromes such as Wilson's disease, the spino-cerebellar degenerations, and idiopathic calcification of the basal ganglia.

The differentiation of these syndromes from the cortical dementias is not always easy. Coincidental development of Alzheimer's disease has been suggested as the explanation for the dementia in Parkinson's disease.

So far, no clear therapeutic advances have arisen from the subdivision.

Investigations

Hb, WBC, ESR (or plasma viscosity), W. R., and HIV antibodies in young at risk groups.

EEG

Can be useful, but normal age changes, e.g. in dominant occipital frequency, may be confusing. Must exclude transient changes due to drug effects, toxic or metabolic disturbances. EEG slowing most common in Alzheimer senile type, positively correlated with cognitive impairment. In early stage may still be normal. Less value in multi-infarct type, unless infarcts large or near surface, when local or focal EEG abnormalities. Creutzfeldt-Jakob disease: slow, disorganised record with periodic complex discharges. May be abnormal sleep patterns in manifest senile dementia.

Results are of greater diagnostic value in patient groups than in individual.

Evoked potentials.
Differential abnormality of the flash compared with pattern visual evoked potentials reported in Alzheimer's disease. Somatosensory evoked potentials more likely to be abnormal in Alzheimer's disease and multi-infarct dementia. As with EEGs, results of greater diagnostic value in patient groups than in the individual.

CT scan
Evidence of atrophy, local or generalised. Degree of ventricular dilatation correlates with severity of dementia.

Combined CT scan and EEG with discriminant analysis can be valuable in Alzheimer's disease.

If necessary to investigate suspected neurological conditions: arteriography, isotope encephalography or in specialised centres MRI scan.

Differential diagnosis of dementia

Depression: may present with complaint of poor concentration and memory, (pseudo dementia). Schizophrenia: simulates dementia through autistic behaviour, self neglect. Hysterical amnesia: global or selective for traumatic events. Chronic drug intoxication: slow, poor concentration (may occur in epileptic patients).

In as many as 31% of patients presumed to be suffering from senile dementia the diagnosis is incorrect, being in fact a depressive illness or an acute confusional state (Ron 1979).

Drug treatment
'Cerebral metabolic enhancers', centrally acting vasodilators, drugs acting at various sites in the cholinergic system, and a miscellaneous group including opioid and adrenergic antagonists, as well as anticonvulsants are all currently suggested as treatment regimens in dementia but have not been shown to have sufficiently sustained benefits to justify their general use outside a research setting.

The amnesic syndromes

Recent memory defect (can register memory but only minimal recall present). May confabulate, confuse temporal sequence of events.

Sudden onset, usually with gradual but incomplete recovery
Bilateral hippocampal infarction (occlusion both posterior cerebral arteries), trauma affecting bilateral medial temporal lobes, subarachnoid haemorrhage, carbon monoxide poisoning.
Traumatic, following a head injury (see separate section, p. 33–35).

Sudden onset, short duration
Complex partial (temporal lobe) seizures. Post-concussion.
'Transient global amnesia', common in the elderly, lasts a few
hours: apparently normal behaviour but slight confusion of vascular
origin (probable transient ischaemia of hippocampal region due to
platelet emboli). Transient during any severe infection, e.g. severe
pneumonia. Local infections: encephalitis, severe meningitis.
Metabolic changes, e.g. cerebral hypoxia, deficiency diseases,
steroids, toxic substances such as carbon monoxide, glue-sniffing,
metallic poisons and drugs, acute alcohol poisoning.

Subacute onset, varying degrees of recovery
Wernicke – Korsakoff syndrome, herpes simplex encephalitis,
tuberculous or other granulomatous basal exudates.

Slowly progressive
Tumours involving floor and walls of third ventricle, early stage of
Alzheimer's disease, other degenerative disorders with
disproportionate involvement of the temporal lobes.

FURTHER READING

Adams, R. D. & Victor, M. (1984) Dementia and the amnesic (Korsakoff)
    syndrome; & Degenerative diseases of the nervous system. In: *Principles
    of Neurology*, pp. 311–321 & 859–901. New York: McGraw Hill.
Byrne, J. & Arie, T. (1985) Rational drug treatment of dementia? *Brit. Med. J.*,
    290, 1845–1846.
Hachinsky, V. C., Lassen, N. A. & Marshall, J. (1974) Multi-infarct dementia. A
    cause of mental deterioration in the elderly. *Lancet*, **ii**, 307–310.
Kasniak, A. W. (1986) The neuropsychology of dementia. In:
    Neuropsychological Assessment of Neuropsychiatric Disorders. ed. Grant,
    I & Adams, K. M. pp. 172–220. Oxford: Oxford University Press.
Katzman, R., Terry, R. D. & Bick, K. L. (1978) Alzheimer's disease: senile
    dementia and related disorders. *Aging*, **Vol. 7**. New York: Raven Press.
Kiloh, L. G. (1975) Psychiatric disturbances of organic origin. *Medicine*, **10**,
    460–468.
Kopelman, M. D. (1987) Amnesia: organic and psychogenic. *Brit. J. Psychiat.*,
    150, 428–443.
Miller, E. (1975) Psychometric assessment. *Brit. J. Hosp. Med.* (Supplement)
    267–272.
Mulley, G. P. (1986) Differential diagnosis of dementia (review article). *Brit.
    Med. J.*, **292**, 1416–1418.
Pearce, J & Miller, D. E. (1973) *Clinical Aspects of Dementia*. London: Balliere
    Tindall.
Roberts, J. K. A. (1984) Dementia. In: *Differential Diagnosis in
    Neuropsychiatry*, pp. 169–191. Chichester: J. Wiley & Son.

Ron, M., Toone, B. E., Garralda, M. E. & Lishman, W. A. (1979) Diagnostic accuracy in presenile dementia. *Brit. J. Psychiat.*, **134**, 161–168.

Roth, M. & Myers, M. H. (1975) The diagnosis of dementia. *Brit. J. Psychiat.*, (Special publication), 87–99.

Roth, M. & Iverson, L. L. (1986) Alzheimer's disease and related disorders. *Brit. Med. Bull.*, **42(1)**, 1–33.

Warrington, E. K. & Gautier-Smith, P. C. (1975) Clinical assessment of higher cerebral function. *Medicine*, **35**, 2049–2053.

C. POST-OPERATIVE PSYCHOSES

INCIDENCE

1 : 1600 surgical operations (severe enough to require psychiatric admission). Increased risk following:

hysterectomy
open heart surgery
cholecystectomy
eye operations.

CAUSES

Metabolic disturbance. Cerebral hypoxia secondary to operative complications such as poor perfusion, cerebral emboli, post-operative sepsis.

Emotional reaction to operation (may be paramount). Withdrawal delirium in alcohol or barbiturate dependent individuals.

CLINICAL VARIANTS

Acute confusional states (when organic factors predominate). Anxiety, depressive or manic states. Schizophrenic psychosis (especially paranoid type).

FURTHER READING

Gath, D. & Day, A. (1982) Hysterectomy and psychiatric disease. *Brit. J. Psychiat.*, **140**, 335–342.

D. PUERPERAL PSYCHOSES

Psychotic illness developing within six months after childbirth.

INCIDENCE

2–3 per 1000 pregnancies. Recurrence rate 20 per 100 subsequent pregnancies.

CAUSES

Usually multifactorial (metabolic and emotional). More common in elderly primiparae, unmarried, previous psychiatric illness, family history of mental illness or difficult pregnancies.

CLINICAL FEATURES

As for post-operative psychoses. Commences abruptly in first two to three weeks, most commonly on third or fourth day after delivery. Initial organic confusional fluctuating disturbance. Later more clearly affective (68%) schizophrenic (27%) or organic (4.5%). May be mixed picture. Outcome tends to be better when affective symptoms predominate. Risk of infanticide high in depressive variants.

DIFFERENTIAL DIAGNOSIS

Puerperal depression

In 10–15% of mothers, onset is usually within a few weeks of delivery, but tends to come to medical attention, if at all, later than does psychosis. Usually lasts a few weeks, but may occasionally become chronic. Dalton blames a fall in levels of circulating progesterone. Pitt has argued that postnatal depression is clinically distinct from classical depressive illness. Watson has found no distinguishing clinical features and suggests that most episodes are explicable in terms of understandable illness in light of previous personality and illness record as well as psychosocial stress.

Maternity blues

Occurs in 50% or more of all mothers. Transient in first few days after childbirth, most commonly 5th day. Ephemeral and resolves without specific treatment.

TREATMENT

Avoid separation if possible (Mother and baby unit). May need physical treatment (phenothiazines and ECT).

FURTHER READING

Dalton, K. (1980) *Depression after childbirth.* Oxford: Oxford University Press.
Kendell, R. E. (1985) Puerperal mental illness. *J. Psychosom. Res.*, **27**, 3–11.
Kumar, R. & Robson, C. K. (1978) *Mental illness in pregnancy and the puerperium*, ed. Sandler, M. Oxford: Oxford Medical Publications.

Pitt, B. (1968) Atypical depression following childbirth. *Brit. J. Psychiat.*, **114**, 1325–1335.

Watson, J. R., Elliott, S. A., Rugg, A. J. & Brough, D. I. (1984) Psychiatric disorder in pregnancy and the first postnatal year. *Brit. J. Psychiat.*, **144**, 453–463.

E. PSYCHIATRIC ASPECTS OF EPILEPSY

ICTUS (the attack)

An occasional, excessive, and disorderly discharge of nerve tissue (Hughlings Jackson).

Types: International Classification of Epileptic Seizures (1981 revision).

I Focal

(Partial, local) May form only the onset (old terminology — aura) or the entire seizure.

A. Simple

No alteration of consciousness.

Motor signs.

Somatosensory or special sensory symptoms or signs.

Autonomic symptoms or signs.

Psychic symptoms, disturbance of higher cerebral function.

B. Complex

Impaired consciousness.

   i. Simple focal onset followed by impaired consciousness
       Similar with automatisms
  ii. Impaired consciousness at the outset, and only impaired consciousness
       Similar with automatisms
 iii. Focal evolving to generalised tonic–clonic convulsions (GTC)
  iv. Simple evolving to GTC
   v. Complex evolving to GTC (including those with simple focal onset).

II Generalised

Convulsive or non-convulsive.

Absence	— typical, regular 3 Hz EEG complex discharges. (6 types — see below).
	— atypical, slow 2 Hz or other polyspike and slow wave EEG complexes.
Myoclonic	— muscle group movements.
Clonic	— whole body movements, multiple jerks of rhythmic or quasi-rhythmic repetition. Distinguished from absence with mild clonic movements on basis of greater duration,

	increased severity, loss of postural tone, slower rate of recovery.
Tonic	— sustained rather than alternating flexor and extensor violent muscular contractions, may be deviation of head, eyes to one side, rotation of the body. Features distorted. If patient aware of these movements then classified as a focal seizure.
Tonic–clonic	— grand mal — sequence of tonic and clonic movements.
Atonic (astatic)	— sudden loss of muscle tone, may be partial, and restricted. Drop attacks. To be differentiated from other types of drop attacks, e.g. transient ischaemia, narcolepsy.

Typical absence seizure types.
  i Impaired consciousness only
  ii With mild tonic–clonic movements
  iii With atonic components. Diminution of muscle tone, often of posture, rarely causing a fall
  iv With tonic components — increased tone, muscle contraction of extensors or flexors. Head movements, retropulsive walking
  v With automatisms, purposeful, semi-purposeful movements in absence of awareness, lip smacking, swallowing, fumbling, aimless walking. Grunting, turning, rubbing site when touched, may be elaborate, or simple
  vi With autonomic components, e.g. changes in respiration, heart rate, pallor, enuresis.

Psychiatric aspects of some of the sub-groups

Psychic symptoms of the simple seizure (1A) types

Dysphasic	— impaired comprehension as well as speech production.
Dysmnesic	— deja and jamais vu — sense of familiarity or unreality in a familiar surround; forced thinking.
Cognitive	— forced thinking, compulsive symptoms, distortions of time sense, dreamy states.
Affective	— emotional expressions, usually unpleasant, e.g. terror, depression, anger, occasionally pleasure, rarely sexual connotation. Ictal rage or anger appears unprovoked, rapidly abates; ictal laughter not accompanied by mirth, not recalled, hence automatism.
Illusions	— sense of distorted visual or auditory perception, derealisation. Depersonalisation.
Hallucinations	— structured, may be also dysmnesic experiences; if simple or crude sensations more likely to be autonomic (focal simple type).

Psychic symptoms of the complex seizure (1B) types
Automatisms — state of clouded consciousness during or
immediately after seizure. Retains control of posture. Performs
simple or complex movements or actions. Lasts < 5 minutes in 80%.
Never > 1 hour. Impaired awareness. Violence rare (< 1%).

In early part of attacks simple oral automatisms, in mid-attack
repetitive more complex stereotyped, picking, pulling, turning.
Some well coordinated patterns — laughing, running; speech
(verbigeration) usually ictal, mid to terminal part of attack. More
elaborate activities seen in post-ictal states, especially after grand-
mal.

In absence seizures oral automatisms occur about 5–6 seconds
after onset, but non-oral occur later. Discharges involve various area
of the limbic system — temporal lobes, cingulate and uncal areas.
Also lesions of frontal and parietal cortex (70–80% incidence in
temporal lobe epilepsy).

POSTICTAL

Automatism.
Confusional psychosis:
 — may be preceded by fits
 — vivid hallucinations
 — delusional ideas (paranoid, religious)
 — may be aggressive if handled tactlessly.

INTERICTAL

Bias in patient selection a major problem in assessing incidence of
various disorders.

No evidence for a specific epileptic personality. Increased risk of
psychological difficulties in major epilepsy and TLE. Reflects site and
extent of any associated brain damage and previous psychosocial
history. Most common when frontal lobes, III ventricular areas
involved. Perseverative/paranoid personality in diffuse brain
damage, bitemporal epilepsy.

Aggressive behaviour. No adequate control study of epileptics
compared with general population.

Prevalence of epilepsy in prison population 7.1/1000 (general
population 4.2/1000).

Violence not more common in epileptic compared with other
prisoners.

In post-traumatic epilepsy, frontal lobe damage predisposes to
aggression and criminality.

Early onset dominant temporal lobe lesion associated with
aggressivity (poor social learning).

Depression. Always a serious matter. Often marked variability —
may be inverse relation to fit frequency. Especially common in
non-dominant temporal lobe lesions.

Suicide. Increased incidence. Access to drugs relevant. Up to 7% life
expectancy of suicide in organic brain disorder with epilepsy.

Dementia. No clear evidence that epilepsy *per se* causes dementia. If
present likely to be due to concomitant organic cerebral disease.
Mimicked by barbiturate over-medication. Prolonged petit mal in
childhood (impairs learning).

Chronic schizophreniform psychosis. Rare. May show any cardinal
symptom of schizophrenia. Often begins long after onset of epilepsy
(median interval 14 years). 65% of cases have TLE.
   May be due to organic temporal lobe lesions (particularly
dominant side). Association between TLE and psychosis regarded
by some as artefact due to patient selection.

Sexual deviation. TLE associated with wide variety of deviant sexual
behaviour (hyposexuality, transvestism, fetishism, homosexuality).
Especially when temporal lobe lesion occurs initially in infancy.

DIAGNOSIS OF EPILEPSY
Primarily clinical, prolonged ambulatory EEG or combined video/
EEG helpful. Eye-witness account. No retrograde amnesia. If an
offence committed it is unpremeditated, usually no attempt made to
conceal.

Differential diagnosis from other psychiatric events

Panic attacks
Acute anxiety, variable form, overwhelming sense of fear or panic.
Long duration (15–30 minutes or more). No change in
consciousness, afterwards all details recalled. May be
hyperventilation. EEG usually no change.

Non-ictal rage or violence
Usually external provocation, may be motive. Attack directional,
amnesia absent or patchy.

Pseudo-seizures, apparent seizures
No electrical brain discharge, EEG no change. Often with an
audience, inappropriate movements, intensified by resistance.
Consciousness preserved, plantars flexor. Exclusion of other

conditions. Separation of hysteria from malingering often impossible. Coexistence of epileptic and pseudo-seizures in the same patient not infrequent.

Fugue state
Syndrome: abrupt loss of personal memory and identity, associated with wandering. Lasts hours or days, with residual amnesia for the period of fugue. Awareness unimpaired.

Causes: Post-ictal confusional states, hypoglycaemia, alcohol intoxication, drugs, transient cerebral ischaemia, transient global amnesia, cerebral tumour. Psychogenic origin not infrequent, with provoking circumstances and gain.

Stress reaction
Episodic aggressive behaviour under stress. May last for hours. Inhibited individuals who use denial mechanisms. No clinical evidence of epilepsy. May be histrionic or depressive element. Rare to injure anyone.

Catatonic schizophrenia
Clear consciousness. Episodic aggressive outbursts. Posturing and stereotyped movements.

Organic confusion
Alcohol, drug intoxication, hypoglycaemia and other metabolic confusional states, infections, cerebral ischaemia, dementia.

Sleep walking
In deep stage IV sleep. Rare to see repetitive stereotyped behaviour. Latter usually well integrated. May need EEG to differentiate sleep state from epilepsy.

AUTOMATISMS AND AGGRESSION

Simple automatisms
Very common in epilepsy, not part of violent and aggressive acts as these require complex movements, interaction with environment.

Complex automatisms
More common in post-ictal confusional states, may be aggressive acts. Usually only pushing, fending-off movements. Only very rarely do complex, directed acts of violence occur.

AUTOMATISMS AND THE LAW

If a patient with epilepsy commit a criminal act, does not realise it, knows the quality and nature of the act but does not appreciate that it is wrong, then he is to be regarded as temporarily insane (according to the McNaughton rules). Thus a patient with epilepsy who commits such an act during an attack is categorised as temporarily insane.

To be differentiated from non-insane automatisms, when someone does something automatically without any conscious exercise of the will. In the latter there is a temporary impairment which results from some external physical factor, e.g. a blow on the head.

FURTHER READING

Fenwick, P. & Fenwick, E. (1985) (eds) *Epilepsy and the Law — A Medical Symposium on the Current Law*. International Congress and Symposium Series. No 81. Royal Society of Medicine.

Laidlaw, J. & Richens, A. (1982) (eds) *A Textbook of Epilepsy*. Edinburgh, London: Churchill Livingstone.

Trieman, D. M. & Delgado-Escueto, A. V. (1983) Violence and Epilepsy: a critical review. In: *Recent Advances in Epilepsy*. eds Pedley, T. A. & Meldrum, B. S. Edinburgh, London: Churchill Livingstone.

Wolf, P. (1985) The classification of seizures and the epilepsies. In: *The Epilepsies*. ed. Porter, R. J. & Morselli, P. L. London: Butterworths.

F. PSYCHIATRIC ASPECTS OF HEAD INJURY

ACUTE EFFECTS

Impaired consciousness

Occurs in all but the mildest closed injuries. Conversely may not occur in localised injury, even if severe and penetrating.
Varying degrees:

   i. Coma — no external evidence of mental activity, little motor activity other than breathing. Depth graded on reflex and EEG activity

  ii. Clouded consciousness — drowsy, incomplete reaction to stimuli. Attention, concentration, memory, orientation impaired

 iii. Confusion — inability to think with speed, clarity and coherence.

Concussion

Closed head injury with momentary loss of consciousness. Usually little or no amnesia, often associated with other features of clouded consciousness. Disorientation, impaired attention and concentration, inability to register or recall events, reduced perception with visual and auditory illusions, or general diminution of all mental activity. May be disordered behaviour, paranoid ideas and hallucinations.

Amnesia

A loss of past memories and inability to form new ones. Can be present with an alert state of mind.

Retrograde — interval between injury and last prior recalled memory. Duration minutes. Poor index of severity or predictor of outcome.

Post-traumatic — PTA — interval between injury and return of normal continuous memory. May be islands of memory — lucid intervals within it. Correlates well with degree of brain damage, and predictive of subsequent outcome, such as cognitive deficits, memory and calculation difficulties, general intellectual impairment, psychiatric and social outcome, personality changes.

Severity of injury judged by amnesic period:

PTA	< 10 min	Very mild injury
PTA	10–60 min	Mild injury
PTA	1–24 h	Moderate injury
PTA	1–7 days	Severe injury
PTA	> 7 days	Very severe injury

< 1 h mild injury

N.B. Other complications, especially infective, can cause toxic confusional states and interfere with assessment of PTA. Older subjects tend to have longer PTAs and more serious deficits for any given PTA. More severe injuries — ability to learn new material is the slowest of cognitive deficits to recover. Pattern of residual deficit resembles Korsakoff amnesic syndrome.

CHRONIC EFFECTS

Related to degree of brain damage, neurological and other sequelae, previous personality, social support, litigation factors.

Cognitive defects

Highly associated with parietal/temporal lobe damage, and degree of tissue loss. Lasting cognitive impairment when PTA > 24 hours.

Affective disorders, personality changes

Associated with frontal lobe injury. May have irritability, loss of drive, disinhibition, aggressive outbursts. Gradual improvement over months or years.

Epilepsy

Incidence about 15% in non-missile, up to 40% in missile. Depends on many factors, principally location, severity, penetration. (Of all patients with epilepsy, 5–15% due to trauma.) Fits most common in the first week after non-missile injury: 27% will be recurrent, only about 20% develop fits later than this, and in these 70% will be recurrent. In missile injuries, one quarter to one third of early onset fits develop late epilepsy, higher incidence with later onset.

Neuroses

Headaches, dizziness, fatigue, irritability, poor concentration, poor memory. No relationship found with brain damage in penetrating injuries. Complex relationship with litigation, compensation. May be perpetuation by focussing anxiety and interest, with conscious or unconscious secondary gain. Recovery after settlement of claim may only occur in a minority (Tarsh and Royston 1985). Over-protective relatives may play a significant perpetuating role; family situation and attitudes need to be assessed in every case.

Post-traumatic encephalopathy (punch drunk syndrome)

Related to extent of exposure to head injury during boxing, usually does not progress after retirement from the ring. Dysartharia, ataxia, slow movements, intellectual impairment, irritability, lack of drive. In some cases morbid jealousy, definite cerebellar, pyramidal, extra-pyramidal signs. X-ray evidence of cerebral atrophy.

CARE OF THE CONFUSED PATIENT

Control of underlying medical disorder, e.g. neurosurgical treatment of haematoma. Quieten patient, protect against injury. Constant vigil, low bed, may need to screen windows, exits. Avoid arousing anxiety or fear, minimal restraint. Only essential drugs, avoid undue sedation. Beware depression of respiration. Control fluids, electrolyte balance, blood pressure, monitor vital function (cardiac, respiratory, neurological). Avoid darkened room, or unnecessary changes of environment. Familiar relative or friend helpful for orientation, contact with reality.

FURTHER READING

Adams, R. D. & Victor, M. (1984) *Principles of Neurology*. 3rd edition. pp. 292–322. New York, McGraw Hill.

Bond, M. R. (1986) Neurobehavioural sequelae of closed head injury. In: *Neuropsychological Assessment of Neuropsychiatric Disorders*. ed. Grant, I. & Adams, K. M. New York, Oxford: Oxford University Press.

Ey, H. (1969) Disorders of consciousness in psychiatry. In: *Handbook of Clinical Neurology*. eds Vinken, P. J. & Bruyn, G. W. Vol. 3. Disorders of Higher Nervous Activity, pp. 112–136. Amsterdam: North Holland.

Kopelman, M. D. (1987) Amnesia: organic and psychogenic. *Brit. J. Psychiat.*, **150**, 428–442.

Lishman, W. A. (1978) *Organic Psychiatry. The Psychological Consequences of Cerebral Disorder*. Oxford: Blackwell.

Roberts, A. H. (1969) *Brain Damage in Boxers*. London: Pitman.

Roberts, J. K. A. (1984) *Differential Diagnosis in Neuropsychiatry*. Chichester: J. Wiley & Sons.

Tarsh, M. J., & Royston, C. (1985) A follow up study of Accident Neurosis. *Brit. J. Psychiat.*, **146**, 18–25.

Trimble, M. F. (1981) *Post Traumatic Neurosis*. Chichester: John Wiley & Sons Ltd.

Psychosomatic disorders

A. OBESITY

ARBITRARY DEFINITION

When body weight exceeds 120% ideal weight for sex, height, medium frame.

PREVALENCE

More common in females, middle age, lower social class.
Females in London:
— age 40–49 years: 30% } are obese
— social class IV–V: 50% }
Children in Buckinghamshire (14-year-olds):
— girls 32.4% } are obese
— boys 3.6% }

CLINICAL FEATURES

Untreated obese individuals show few neurotic traits.
Obese patients have Increased incidence of emotional difficulties.
Social stereotype leads to scapegoating and exclusion especially in childhood. Predisposes to denial, self loathing and over-estimate of body size.

NEUROLOGICAL SUBSTRATE

Energy homeostasis achieved by balance between ventromedial and lateral hypothalamic nuclei (hunger and satiety centres). These under influence of internal cues (metabolic) and external cues (palatability of foods, learnt attitude to food).

CAUSES

Predisposing
Psychological factors less obvious in late onset type.
Genetic. MZ twins high concordance for body weight.

Developmental. Increased total fat cell number through overfeeding in childhood. Aberrant family attitudes to food: substitute for comfort, obesity equated with well-being.

Precipitating
Emotional upset may lead to obesity in predisposed individuals because eating causes tension release.

TREATMENT
High default and relapse rate, variable motivation.
1. *Diet.* Dietary (calorie) restriction over extended period.
2. *Psychological.* Extended individual/group support. Dieting may lead to irritability, depression, loss of denial defence. Conjoint therapy with spouse (deal with factors preventing dieting in family situation).
3. *Drugs.* Anorectics: use intermittently (danger of dependence). Phentermine and chlorphentermine useful in lethargic depressed patients. Fenfluramine a central anorectic with peripheral effect on glucose uptake. May lead to depression on withdrawal. Useful in the anxious and overactive.
4. *Surgical adjuncts.* Jaw wiring: useful in initiating weight loss when all else fails.
   Ileojejunostomy: increased assertiveness and sexual interest. Family adjustment difficulties may follow. May be up to 25% incidence of post-operative depression and suicidal ideas. Persistent diarrhoea and electrolyte disturbance, impaired liver function: gastric plication a recent development.

FURTHER READING

Garrow, J. S. (1981) *Treat Obesity Seriously: A Clinical Manual.* Edinburgh: Churchill Livingstone.
Kalucy, R. S. (1977) Obesity. In *Modern Trends in Psychosomatic Medicine*, **3**, 404–429.

B. ANOREXIA NERVOSA

First described independently by Sir William Gull (1868) and Lasegue (1873).
Females outnumber males 15:1 (case register data).
Most common in upper social classes.
Average age onset 15.5 years (87% within 5 years of menarche).
Point prevalence: 1% girls age 16–18 years in private schools.
1–2% of female university students.
Minor variants in community more common than severe cases.
Recent increased incidence likely, especially in less severe form.

CLINICAL FEATURES

1. Physical

Marked loss of body weight and malnutrition due to:
— purposive avoidance of 'fattening foods', self induced vomiting.
— purgation, excessive exercise, use of diuretics, subterfuges in disposal of food.

Nutritional myopathy (gross muscle wasting with good power and brisk tendon reflexes).

Bradycardia, cold extremities with peripheral cyanosis, normal secondary sexual hair, episodic bulimia.

The patient claims to feel well, and is often physically very active.

Usually apyrexial, normal white blood cell count and plasma viscosity. If these are abnormal then some complication is likely.

2. Endocrine

Specific hypothalamic-hypophyseal failure of gonadotrophin secretion. In females: amenorrhoea may precede or coincide with weight loss in 50%, and so it is not necessarily explicable as being secondary to it.

In males: Loss of sexual interest, impotence.

Low oestrogen, testosterone, LH, gonadotrophin. Euthyroid. Raised GH and cortisol. Delayed return of cyclical gonadotrophin output from pituitary when weight returns to normal.

3. Psychological

a. Marked fear of becoming fat (Russell): phobia for normal body weight (Crisp). Explicit or implicit in behaviour. Strives to be thin, believes self to be fat when thin; loss of judgement concerning food requirements, sets weight limits below normal.

b. Non-specific.
   Depression 25–50%, obsessional symptoms 20–25%, anxiety 40%.
   Highly conscientious, strives to achieve.
   Extremely rigid thinking, stubbornly adheres to self imposed dietary regime. Resents and is angered as well as made anxious by intervention aimed at increasing body weight. Shoplifting (especially items of food). Overvalued control of the self.

CAUSES AND PSYCHODYNAMICS

The psychobiological regression hypothesis suggests that anorexia nervosa is a state of regression (triggered by nutritional deprivation) which then allows phobic avoidance of personal conflict. Puberty is a weight-related event, signalled by the passing of a threshold body weight: patients with anorexia nervosa have a neuroendocrine state which resembles pre-puberty. Loss of weight may be rewarding and liable to lead to anorexia nervosa in certain vulnerable adolescents (those who are experiencing difficulties with the transitions inherent in adolescence), because the biological regression which it brings leads also to psychological regression (loss of libido) or emancipation (invalidism). This process of 'switching off' tends to be self perpetuating because the individual fears weight gain with return of conflicts. Deliberate dieting (common in adolescent females) is therefore at risk of precipitating anorexia nervosa in a small proportion of vulnerable individuals who embark upon it. Early menarche may similarly act as precipitant.

Family factors may be important: increased incidence of marital difficulties in parents and psychiatric illness in mother: high parental expectation of achievement (both in themselves and their children). Minuchin claims specific pattern of enmeshment, overprotection, rigidity, lack of conflict resolution. The anorexic illness may sometimes serve the purpose of keeping the family together. 6–10% of female siblings of patients with anorexia nervosa also have this illness.

No demonstrable organic disorder of hypothalamus, although occasionally hypothalamic tumours can cause severe disorder of food intake and marked weight loss.

DIFFERENTIAL DIAGNOSIS

Malabsorption syndrome, Crohn's disease, reticulosis, diabetes mellitus, thyrotoxicosis, gastro-intestinal neoplasia.

Depressive illness, phobic anxiety state, obsessional neurosis, paranoid psychosis (with fears of food being poisoned).

Bulimia nervosa characterised by intractable urges to overeat (often leading to 'binge' episodes of massive food intake), use of self induced vomiting and/or purgatives to avoid the fattening effects of food. There is also a characteristic fear of becoming fat. Bulimia nervosa may be unsuspected because body weight is often near normal. It may be much more common than anorexia nervosa (although 35–50% of patients with bulimia nervosa go through a state which is identical with anorexia nervosa). Note also anorexia nervosa is complicated by binge eating in up to 50% of cases (see below).

COMPLICATIONS

Physical

Oedema, impaired excretion of water load (especially in chronic illness). Electrolyte disturbance, e.g. hypokalemia, alkalosis (gross muscle weakness with absent reflexes), alkalosis due to persistent vomiting. Tetany, secondary to extreme alkalosis and its effect on ionised calcium (muscle spasm, main accoucheur, stridor which may lead to severe dyspnoea, generalised paraesthesiae).

Dehydration. Secondary hyperaldosteronism.
Hypercholesterolaemia. Carotenaemia. Hypoglycaemia.
Hypothermia. Moderate normochromic normocytic anaemia, Hb
10–11 g%. (Occasionally aplastic crisis.)
  Follicular hyperkeratosis. Lanugo type hair on trunk.
  Life threatening inanition when weight loss falls to the region of
50% expected.

Psychological
Intense family reaction (anxiety, hostility, wish to control). Aversion
to food worse when weight loss severe. Reactive depression and
suicide risk.

Iatrogenic
Phenothiazines (epileptic fits, jaundice).
Tricyclic antidepressants (epileptic fits, cardiac arrhythmias,
deliberate self overdosage).

Treatment
Two main aims:
  1. Restoration of adequate nutrition. This may be an urgent
requirement. Admission to hospital imperative if body weight is in
the region of 60% or less of average. Admit earlier if weight loss is
rapid, especially if dehydration and electrolyte imbalance are
significant.
  2. Resolution of underlying psychosocial causes. Treatment
programmes vary. Both Russell and Crisp emphasise importance of
restoration of adequate weight gain without delay. This usually
requires admission to hospital, sometimes initially with bed rest.
Rationale: weight increase allows the weight phobia to be tackled
and it triggers the return of normal endocrine function, setting the
scene for restoration of normal sexual feelings. Stonehill
recommends a treatment contract involving weight gain of 3–4
pounds a week, a non-negotiable target weight, bed rest, 3000
calories per day. Restlessness is treated with chlorpromazine.
Psychotherapy is aimed at rekindling feelings, and family dynamics
should also be addressed.
  Other approaches (Morgan et al) emphasise out-patient therapy,
more gradual weight gain, extended close psychotherapeutic
alliance involving, where possible, the same therapist over an
extended period. Each step is negotiated with the patient: the
therapist is supportive but also firm. Early intervention may be
important in determining good outcome.
  Physical complications may need treatment and their prevention
is an important element in the treatment programme. Depression
may reach suicidal intensity, especially if weight gain is rapid.
Antidepressant medication should be used with caution, particularly
when electrolyte disturbance is present. In some cases ECT may

have to be used. Rarely feeding through nasoesophageal tube has to be used, but this should always be in an atmosphere of persuasion rather than forceful intervention. Rapid weight gain by this means may precipitate very severe psychological upset, sometimes with paranoid ideas and suicidal motivation. In extreme weight loss a patient who is unable to cooperate with treatment and who is at great physical risk may require compulsory treatment under a section of The Mental Health Act.

Anxiolytics and antidepressants when symptomatically indicated. (High doses of chlorpromazine recommended by some.)

Recent research suggests that family therapy has distinct advantages over individual therapy in younger patients (less than 17 years). In older patients, individual therapy may be equally effective.

LONG TERM OUTCOME

Body weight has to be maintained near normal for some time before menstruation returns.

Follow-up studies should be at least 5 years in duration in order to allow for recovery from initial illness. Precise outcome depends on case selection. The following represents out come findings based on hospital-referred patients.

Normal weight and menstruation: 39–58%
Intermittent weight loss, menstrual abnormality: 19–30%
Constant low weight (85% a.b.w.) and amenorrhoea: 19–29%
Death: 1–5% (severe weight loss, suicide, gross electrolyte disorder such as hypokalaemia leading to ileus, intestinal distention and perforation, infection or septicaemia, iatrogenic such as drug toxic side effects).

PROGNOSTIC FACTORS

Poor outcome when illness prolonged, late onset (19 years or older), previous childhood adjustment difficulties, poor relationship with family.

C. BULIMIA NERVOSA

CLINICAL FEATURES

Females greatly outnumber males (approx. 1–2% of young women). Age onset late teenage and early twenties. 12% of females and 6% of males in college populations admit to self induced vomiting. May be weight normalised anorexia nervosa (in less than 50%) 50% have amenorrhoea. Loss of control of food intake: powerful intractible urges to over-eat, leading to episodic binges associated with great distress and loss of control.

Body weight remains within normal limits.

Self-induced vomiting and/or abusive purgatives.

Marked fear of becoming fat.

In DSMIII the syndrome of bulimia specifically excludes anorexia nervosa, and places emphasis on the presence of depression with self deprecatory thoughts, especially subsequent to binge episodes. May be chaotic pattern of food intake, with spells of starvation for days on end following each binge/vomit episode. Such erratic food intake may be an important perpetuating factor, maintaining chronicity of the illness.

Vomiting is often induced by pushing fingers into pharynx: physical trauma may lead to callosities on dorsa of hands.

Clinical sub-groups (Lacey):

— neurotic (the majority). Hard working and ambitious. Give superficial impression of coping well. Depressive features and anger, with low self esteem. Anxiety and phobic features as well as depersonalisation also may occur.

— personality disordered (the minority). Food difficulties are associated with similar disordered intake of alcohol and drug abuse. Brief bouts of pathological drinking or drug abuse may be interspersed with periods of abstinence. Deliberate self harm common.

COMPLICATIONS

Gross electrolyte imbalance (hypokalaemic alkalosis), dehydration.

Depression, suicidal ideas.

Erosion of dental enamel by acid gastric juices.

Bilateral painless swelling of parotid salivary glands (mechanism unknown).

CAUSES

Probably a relatively new syndrome which has increased rapidly in prevalence during the last 20 years. Aetiology poorly understood, but may include social pressures on females toward dietary restraint. Patients have significantly increased personal and family history of obesity. In some the causal factors relevant to anorexia nervosa are important.

Background or precipitating problems include relationship difficulties, parental conflict, academic striving, loss events.

Perpetuation: a binge may lead to reduction of tension at first, with initial feeling of relief.

TREATMENT

Aims to reduce the frequency and severity of binge episodes. A variety of approaches may be used:
- education regarding dangers of vomiting/purgation and the physiology of hunger, fasting, eating
- regularisation of food intake. Keep a diary recording binge episodes, associated events and feelings. Establish regular mealtimes, avoid periods of starvation
- ritualise the binge episodes. Emphasise alternative pleasurable behaviours
- relaxation techniques and anxiety management
- depressive symptoms may require antidepressant medication
- cognitive behaviour therapy (Fairburn)
- group psychotherapy (Lacey)

FURTHER READING

Crisp, A. H. (1980) *Anorexia Nervosa: Let Me Be.* London: Academic Press.
Fairburn, C. (1982) *Binge-eating and Bulimia Nervosa.* Smith Kline & French publications. Vol 1 No 4.
Lacey, J. H. (1985) Time Limited and Group Treatment for Bulimia. *In Handbook of Psychotherapy for Anorexia Nervosa and Bulimia.* ed. Garner, D. M. and Garfinkel, P. E. London: The Guildford Press.
Morgan, H. G. (1982) Anorexia nervosa. *Practitioner,* **226**, 1941–1947.
Morgan, H. G. et al. (1983) Management and outcome in anorexia nervosa. *Brit. J. Psychiat.,* **143**, 282–287.
Morgan, H. G. (1985) Functional vomiting. *J. Psychosom. Res.,* **29**, 341–352.
Palmer, R. L. (1980) *Anorexia Nervosa.* Harmondsworth: Penguin Books.
Russell, G. F. M. R. (1987) Anorexia nervosa and bulimia nervosa. *The Oxford Text Book of Medicine.* Oxford Medical Publications.

D. PSYCHOGENIC VOMITING

CLINICAL FEATURES AND CAUSES

Persistent and recurrent vomiting in the absence of any other demonstrable cause.
Remittent pattern over months or years.
Females outnumber males 5:1. Usually young/middle-aged adults.
History of vomiting in childhood common.
Severity of clinical picture varies with case selection.
Rosenthal (outpatient clinic): stress related syndrome of relatively good prognosis with trivial weight loss.
Hill (inpatients in general hospital): chronic disabling syndrome with significant weight loss and electrolyte disturbance. Unresolvable relationship problems common, low assertiveness, passive dependency.

TREATMENT

Attention to precipitating stress factors. Anxiety control management. Psychotherapeutic approach relevant to individual or relationship difficulties. Caution in use of anxiolytic medication because of risk of dependence. May require antidepressant medication. Behavioural therapy techniques can be useful. Modification of feeding patterns may influence vomiting in the mentally handicapped.

FURTHER READING

Morgan, H. G. (1985) Functional vomiting. *J. Psychosom. Res.* **29**, 341–352.

E. ASSESSMENT OF PAIN

DEFINITION

Pain is an unpleasant experience which we primarily associate with tissue damage, or describe in terms of such damage or both (Merskey).

PAIN OF PSYCHOLOGICAL ORIGIN

May be: 1. Continuous for long periods by day.
2. Tends not to be the subject of sharp accentuation.
3. Is often recognised by patients as having emotional precipitants.
4. May prevent getting off to sleep but not cause wakening.

PSYCHOLOGICAL MECHANISMS

1. Influence severity and character of pain due to organic disorder.
2. May perpetuate pain when organic cause has resolved.
3. Can produce pain in absence of organic disease.
   Those which influence pain perception include:

Aggression (arousal and distraction): reduction of pain sensation (battle injuries).
Anxiety/depression: increased pain perception. May present as 'pain problem'.
Schizophrenia: delusional ideas of passivity or bizarre hypochondriasis.
Hysterical conversion.
Malingering.
Identification: bereavement or commonly some painful illness in relative.

ASSESSMENT OF PAIN PROBLEM

(When organic disease is judged absent or trivial).
Both organic and psychological factors may be present. Need to interview several informants. Aim to get consistent positive psychological evidence from several sources.

Family. Ethnic variation in attitudes, bereavement, current illness, wife pregnant (Couvade syndrome).

Previous personality. Attitudes to illness and tolerance of painful conditions. Hypochondriasis. Mood variation. Situational vulnerabilities.

Previous psychiatric illness. May resemble current symptoms in quality, cause, course.

Life situation. Recent stress, especially those to which vulnerable. Litigation.

The symptoms. Bizarre quality not necessarily indicative of psychogenic cause.

TREATMENT

Beware of escalation in use of sedatives and analgesics. Patients with psychogenic pain often hostile to psychological approach.

FURTHER READING

Merskey, H. (1980) Psychiatry and the treatment of pain. *Brit. J. Psychiat.,* **136**, 600–602.

F. ISCHAEMIC HEART DISEASE (IHD)

BEHAVIOURAL TYPES

A proposed causal link between psychosocial factors and IHD. Implies that inappropriate emotional reaction to stress predisposes to IHD.

Type A characteristics: impatience, sense of urgency, competitiveness, aggressiveness, hyperalertness, explosive speech, abruptness of gesture. Not a personality type, but a constellation of behaviour manifested under particular circumstances by susceptible individuals. Can be measured reliably using Rosenman's structured interview, recently developed in videotape form.
Type B characteristics: the absence of these behavioural features.

CAUSAL MECHANISMS

Increased incidence of IHD in Type A men (cross sectional and longitudinal studies). Causal factors may involve more rapid blood clotting, increased platelet aggregation in Type A individuals.
In the Western Collaborative Project and Framlingham studies (USA) a positive association was found even after controlling for other risk factors such as cigarette smoking, blood pressure and serum cholesterol. Recent studies in the UK confirm these findings concerning coronary heart disease but not for the subsequent incidence of myocardial infarction.
The twentieth century 'epidemic' of IHD may be due to increased prevalence of Type A behaviour (Rosenman), but other complex aetiological factors also likely.
Risk in Type A is twice that in Type B.
Type A behaviour may be most useful in predicting high risk when combined with other risk factors: when present with hypertension the risk of IHD may be 6% over 2½ years.
Conversely, Type B individuals with low serum lipids and lipoproteins may constitute a low risk group.
  Conflicting research findings may be due to systematic bias in patient selection (angina or myocardial infarction, hospitalised or not, self-exclusion from studies, Type A patients more likely to demand investigation).
  Association is not necessarily of causal significance, and intervention studies are needed. Friedman reports that reduction of Type A behaviour through counselling after myocardial infarction leads to reduction in subsequent cardiac morbidity.

PSYCHOLOGICAL ASPECTS OF ACUTE IHD

Distress and disability may be more related to psychological and social problems than to organic symptoms themselves.

CONCOMITANTS

About 50% of IHD patients have high levels of anxiety and/or depression in between acute episodes of illness, and emotional precipitants of angina include anger, excitement or anxiety (Mayou). Denial is a significant defence mechanism in 60% of IHD patients: in some it may interfere with management by reducing treatment compliance.

SECONDARY DISABILITY

Irritability
Secondary family problems in 70%. Relatives anxious, overprotective or resentful, avoidance of sexual relationship.

Only a minority discontinue *alcohol intake, smoking*.
Return to work less common in those who had previous personality difficulties and such patients exhibit greater emotional upset during acute IHD. Patients with mild angina tend to remain off work longer than those with severe IHD.

MANAGEMENT

Planned integrated team approach allows effective and prompt attention to be paid to physical, psychological and social factors concurrently.

Emotional wellbeing closely related to adequate reassurance, explanation, management of defence reactions, control of affective disturbance both in patient and relatives.

FURTHER READING

Editorial (1980) Type A behaviour and ischaemic heart disease. *Psychological Medicine*, **10**, 603–608.
Mayou, R. (1973) The patient with angina. *Postgrad. Med. J.*, **49**, 250–254.
Sensky, T. (1987) Leading article. Refining thinking on Type A behaviour and coronary heart disease. *Brit. Med. J.*, **295**, 69–70.

The schizophrenias

1. DEVELOPMENT OF CONCEPT AND DIAGNOSTIC DEFINITIONS

Emil Kraepelin (*1896*). Dementia praecox implied deterioration during course of illness. Grouped under this rubric-catatonic, hebephrenic and paranoid states. Later added category of 'simple' schizophrenia.

Eugene Bleuler (*1911*). Fundamental disorder involved splitting of psychological functions. Coined term 'schizophrenias': deterioration not inevitable, the content and meaning of psychotic symptoms were emphasised. Concept of fundamental versus accessory symptoms.

Adolf Meyer (*1910*). Psychobiological school. Saw schizophrenia as a reaction to traumatic life situation. Insisted on unique, idiosyncratic response in each individual, and eschewed general rules of psychodynamics.

ICD9 defines schizophrenic psychoses as that group of illnesses in which there is a fundamental disturbance of personality, a characteristic disorder of thinking, often a sense of being controlled by alien forces, delusions which may be bizarre, disturbed perception, abnormal affect out of keeping with the real situation, and autism. The diagnosis should not be restricted to conditions running a protracted, deteriorating or chronic course. Delineates the following types: simple, hebephrenic, catatonic, paranoid, acute, latent, residual and schizoaffective (see ICD9 for details).

DSMIII of the A.P.A. adopts a cross-sectional and longitudinal approach under six headings:
A. Characteristic symptoms and behaviour (delusions, hallucinations, thought disorder, behaviour).
B. Deterioration from a previous level of functioning in such areas as work, social relations, self-care.
C. Duration: continuing signs of illness for at least 6 months at any time (if less, but more than 2 weeks, then diagnosis becomes schizophrenic disorder).
D. Any affective symptoms develop secondary to other psychotic features, and brief in duration.

48

E. Onset of prodromic or active phase of illness before age of 45 years.
F. Not due to an organic mental disorder or mental retardation.

2. PHENOMENOLOGY

Delusions

Present in 71%.

Primary (autochthonous): not understandable in terms of preceding morbid experience. Sudden onset. Delusional perception when abnormal significance is attached to normal perception which is accorded a sense of urgent importance. Often self referring.

Secondary: arise out of some other morbid experience, e.g. persecutory delusions relating to hallucinations.

Delusions may be related to morbid ideas of passivity (influence or control by an outside agency) e.g. thought insertion or withdrawal, or being made to think. Distinguish from 'as if' experiences which lack delusional conviction.

Thought disorder

Low consistency between constructs (Kelly Repertory Grid).
Over-inclusive, asyndetic, imprecise, interpenetrating themes (Cameron).
Concrete thinking, impaired abstract thought (Goldstein).
Peripheral and irrelevant features of a total concept assume central significance. Thinking becomes vague, elliptical and obscure, and speech may be incoherent. Breaks in the flow of consecutive thought are frequent. Mood may be shallow or incongruous. Ambivalence may appear as inertia, negativism or stupor. Catatonia may be present: this is a psychomotor disturbance, often alternating between extremes such as hyperkinesis and stupor, or automatic obedience and negativism. Limbs may remain in fixed placed positions for long periods. May be severe excitement.

Hallucinations

Form: auditory 95%, visual 30%, less commonly olfactory, tactile, bodily, gustatory.
Content: usually voices of relatives or other familiar figures.
Threatening in 33%. May comment on the patient or address him.

Schneider's first rank symptoms

Can be reliably detected and defined clearly. Present in 28–72% of schizophrenic illnesses.

Claimed to be diagnostic when one or more present, in absence of organic brain disease or other relevant pathology. Important to remember that their significance can only be assessed in the light of the total clinical picture, previous personality and cultural background. Great caution in assessment when severe depression or manic elevation of mood present.

The first rank symptoms are:
a. Audible thoughts.
b. Voices arguing, running commentary on patient's actions.
c. Somatic passivity: experiences of physical interference by outside influences.
d. Thought withdrawal, insertion or interruption by outside influence.
e. Thought broadcasting, or believe others to think the same thoughts.
f. Delusional perception.
g. Feelings, impulses, volitional acts thought to be due to others.

First rank symptoms have no theoretical value and have poor prognostic significance. May occur in 13% of mania, 15% depressive disorders, 2% neuroses. Variation in assessment of specificity and validity may be due to inadequate interview method. Careful and extended clinical interview required, based on phenomenological technique, in order to demonstrate first rank symptoms reliably.

Bleuler's fundamental symptoms
Loosened associations between psychological functions, autism, ambivalence, disorders of affect.

These are not easy to detect in a reliable way.

Variation in diagnostic fashion
Concept of schizophrenia is wider in the USA, where in some parts (New York) it is diagnosed twice as often as in Europe.

Incidence
Illness expectancy 15–45 years = 0.5–1%.
First admissions to hospital 15–20/100 000 per annum.

Clinical types
Hebephrenic: *onset*   15–25 years. Thought disorder, incongruous affect.
Catatonic: 15–40 years. Motor disorders.? Becoming less common.
Paranoid: 15–60 years. Delusional ideas (with or without hallucinations).
Simple: Young adult. Loss of drive, social deterioration. Delusions and hallucinations not evident. May end in vagrancy. Dubious entity.

Good prognostic indicators
Acute onset, obvious precipitating stress.
Good previous personality, strong affective component.
Described by Langfeldt (1939) as schizophreniform psychoses.
Well-preserved affect, paranoid (less likely to deteriorate).

Poor prognostic indicators
Onset before 20 years, schizoid previous personality, insidious
onset, hebephrenic type, family history of deteriorating
schizophrenia. This type of clinical picture has been termed 'nuclear'
or 'process' type.
    Poor outcome associated with prominent negative symptoms in
first illness (blunted affect, poverty of speech, social withdrawal)
(Kolakowska et al).

3. CLINICAL COURSE

Five years follow-up period (Wing)
Chronic: symptoms throughout	28%
episodic	27%
Improving: well in last 2½ years	11%
Acute: symptoms limited to first year	34%

4. SOCIAL OUTCOME

At 5 years (Wing)
In hospital during whole of 5-year period	11%
Severely disturbed in last 6 months	17%
Minor symptoms only: not working	16%
working	7%
Well and self-supporting	49%

Enormous improvement in proportion requiring long term
hospitalisation in recent decades (60% → 11%), but not much
change in proportion which show symptoms.
    Similar findings from more recent study of a representative
sample of patients in Buckinghamshire (Watts et al 1983), in which
48% of cohort and 58% of first admissions had good outcome after 5
years. Females did better than males.
    Manfred Bleuler suggests that advances in pharmacological and
psychosocial treatments have greatly benefitted patients with
fluctuating illness, but have had little effect on incidence of illness
which remits with little deficit, or fail to respond at all.

5. SOCIAL CORRELATES

Prevalence more common in social class V (likely to be due to social
drift because social class of fathers no different from expectation).
    Prognosis worse in social class V.

Social handicaps

Primary: Due to florid symptoms.

Secondary: Changed attitudes of others, loss of social contacts, impaired drive, general indifference (all worse with prolonged stay in hospital).

Other: Poverty, lack of education, deprived of family support.

6. THE 'NEW LONG STAY' HOSPITAL PATIENTS (Mann & Cree)

In 1971, 21% of mental hospital patients had been there 1–5 years, of these 44.4% were schizophrenic.

7. SOME SIMILAR BUT DISTINCT CONDITIONS: ICD9 DEFINITIONS

Paranoid psychosis

Acute or chronic illness, not classifiable as schizophrenia or affective psychosis, in which delusions, especially of being influenced, persecuted or treated in some special way, are the main symptoms. The delusions are of a fairly fixed, elaborate and systematised kind.

Paranoia

A rare chronic psychosis in which logically constructed systematised delusions have developed gradually without concomitant hallucinations or the schizophrenia type of disordered thinking. The delusions are mostly of grandeur (the paranoiac prophet or inventor), persecution or somatic abnormality.

Paraphrenia

A paranoid psychosis in which there are conspicuous hallucinations, often in several modalities. Affective symptoms and disordered thinking, if present, do not dominate the clinical picture and the personality is well preserved.

This syndrome is sometimes developed in the elderly, especially single, socially isolated females who have sensory deficit such as deafness.

8. AETIOLOGICAL THEORIES

Family environment

(Bateson) Parent-child relationship. Double bind communications involving incompatible opposites. Forced to decide between alternatives both of which are disapproved. Child forced into inactivity or ambiguous response.

(Lidz) Whole family pathology. Close relationship with parent of opposite sex. Family dominated by the relationship. Other parent withdrawn, inadequate (skew). Hostile relationship in family (schism).

(Wynne and Sanger) Family communication resembles schizophrenic psychopathology: fragmented, undirected. Possible to differentiate families of schizophrenic patients from normals in double blind control situation.

(Laing) Schizophrenogenic mother: close, engulfing, exclusive, overprotective, ambivalent. Prevents maturation in child which doubts own feelings and sense of identity.

Other family processes: blurred generation lines, psychological abnormalities of various kinds in first degree relatives, increased incidence of parental loss before 10 years.

Biochemical

Defect of amines and aminergic transmission. Functional excess or deficiency of amines involved in CNS transmission, or production of abnormal metabolites: due to error in metabolic pathway or variation in receptor sensitivity. Critique: uncertain whether toxic metabolites cause symptoms specifically analogous to those of schizophrenia. Difficult to control for metabolic changes caused by chronic hospitalisation.

Indoleamine metabolism. Reduction of available serotonin may be basis for reserpine induced improvement in schizophrenia.

Bad LSD 'trip' may resemble schizophrenia. Note that LSD affects serotonin-containing neurones and antagonises serotonin in vitro.

Methylated indoles can be psychotomimetic. There may be increased excretion of methylated indoles during relapse of schizophrenia.

Catecholamine metabolism. Adrenaline normally synthesised from phenylalanine via dopamine. Possible error of phenylalanine or adrenaline metabolism (oxidation, methylation). May be error of dopaminergic transmission.

Adrenaline

Dopamine

5 Hydroxytryptamine (Serotonin)

Mescaline

Methylated catecholamines can be psychotomimetic. The hallucinogen mescaline (dimethoxyphenylethylamine) might be derived from dopamine.

Strong case that antipsychotic effects of neuroleptic drugs are due to block of postsynaptic dopamine receptors. Also evidence of abnormality of dopaminergic transmission in some schizophrenic patients. Post-mortem studies have reported increase in both dopamine and dopamine receptors in the caudate nucleus, the nucleus accumbens and the limbic areas in schizophrenic patients. Some parkinsonian patients on high dose L dopa treatment develop psychotic reactions. Amphetamine (which releases dopamine at central synapses) induces a disorder indistinguishable from schizophrenia, and worsens schizophrenic symptoms. Although antipsychotic drugs may act by blocking dopamine receptors, there is still no specific evidence that abnormality of dopamine metabolism is of causal significance in schizophrenia.

Crow points out that dopamine hypothesis is of restricted application: neuroleptic drugs are of limited value in many chronic patients, who are also often resistant to the exacerbating effects of dexamphetamine which increases dopamine release. Suggests two distinct schizophrenic syndromes reflecting different pathological process: one characterised by 'positive' and the other by 'negative' symptoms.

	Syndrome I	*Syndrome II*
Symptoms	Positive (delusions, hallucinations, thought disorder)	Negative (affective flattening, poverty of speech, loss of volition)
Most common	in acute schizophrenia	in chronic schizophrenia
Potential response to neuroleptic drugs	good	poor
Intellectual impairment	absent	sometimes present (correlates with increased ventricular size on CAT scan)
Outcome	reversible	? irreversible
Pathological process	increased dopamine receptors (post-mortem evidence)	cell loss and structural brain changes, possibly encephalitic process

Mackay suggests that Syndromes I and II are both based on instability in control of dopaminergic transmission. Type I: overactivity, Type II: underactivity.

Genetic
1. Frequency of schizophrenia greater in families of patients than in controls. Life expectancy gen. pop'n. 0.9%, first degree relatives (parents, children, siblings) 10–14%; second degree relatives (uncles, aunts, grandparents, grandchildren) 3–7%; MZ twins 35–80%; DZ twins 10%; children of two affected parents 35–50%. Variation in some degree related to clinical severity, early onset (both increase risk) or paranoid illness, antecedent organic cerebral illness (both reduce risk).
2. Adult schizophrenics born of hospitalised schizophrenic mothers adopted at birth: 16.6% developed schizophrenia compared with none in controls (Heston, USA).
3. Extended family study: excess of schizophrenic spectrum disorders in biological relatives of adopted adults who become schizophrenic (Kety, Denmark).
4. Adoptees with schizophrenic parent showed schizophrenic spectrum disorders twice as often as did controls (Rosenthal, Denmark).
5. Adoptive parent study: biological parents showed more psychological disturbance than adoptive parents of schizophrenics (Wender, USA).

Possible genetic mechanisms. Schizophrenics probably genetically heterogenous. Genetic predisposition interacts with environmental trigger. Polygenic theory is currently most popular (Gottesman and Shields). This accounts for threshold effects, gradation of severity, importance of non-genetic aetiological factors.

Murray et al. (see Wing) suggest genetic and non-genetic variations of schizophrenia, the latter being more likely to be associated with enlarged ventricles and a history of environmental damage.

Environmental
Sharp increase in number of life events, some independent of patient's behaviour during three weeks prior to onset of acute illness. Most kinds of life events may trigger onset or relapse, often associated with stopping phenothiazine medication. Relapse less likely in situations of low emotional involvement and with work appropriate to capacity.

9. TREATMENT

Physical

Drugs
Phenothiazines. (Leff 1972) If maintained for one year after remission, 33% relapse compared with 83% controls. (Double blind design study of acute schizophrenia.)

I.m. long acting preparations over nine month period: 8% relapsed compared with 66% placebo controls (may be effective when oral medication poorly absorbed: may precipitate severe depression in predisposed individuals: tardive dyskinesia). Avoidance of maintenance therapy may be justified if first illness with good prognostic signs.

Drugs may delay relapse but do not necessarily prevent it. Johnson reports in 2 years 41% relapse, and 33% may be drug non-responders.

Low dosage maintenance therapy has recently been proposed: even though relapse rate may be greater than with conventional dosage, symptoms may be less severe, response to therapy good and fewer long term side effects such as tardive dyskinesia (Hirsch 1986).

Stopping drug treatment (Drug and Therapeutics Bulletin 1987). Treatment over a 3-year period with antipsychotic drugs reduces the risk of relapse 3-fold compared with placebo. Unwanted effects of maintenance treatment include mental fatigue, lethargy, akathisia, dystonic reactions and parkinsonian movement disorders. Approximately 15–20% of patients on prolonged treatment may develop tardive dyskinesia, which often persists after drugs stopped. Withdrawal of drugs is a difficult decision. Probable that in established schizophrenia the advantages of continuing long term antipsychotic medication outweigh the disadvantages. Withdrawal should only be considered in a patient with a stable social environment who has had no psychotic symptoms for at least 6 months, who can recognise early signs of relapse and is likely to accept resumption of drug therapy.

Drug withdrawal should be done gradually over several months and monitored carefully.

Two types of withdrawal syndromes, though uncommon if dose reduction is gradual.

Acute: within a few days, nausea, vomiting, diarrhoea, restlessness, insomnia, rhinorrhoea — may be due to cholinergic overactivity.

Withdrawal dyskinesias: arise de novo, or worsening of pre-existing disorder. Most remit within a few weeks.

Thioxanthines. I.m. flupenthixol decanoate may be less likely to cause depression.

ECT
Not superior to drug therapy, but together with them may possibly lead to more rapid improvement.

Social
Manipulation of social forces with intention of reducing symptoms. Relapse more likely when return to situations with high emotional and critical expressiveness and closeness (high expressed emotion, HEE). Counselling of relatives and patient may lessen relapse rate, especially when combined with drug treatment (Vaughn and Leff 1976). A controlled 2-year follow-up study of social intervention in families of schizophrenic patients in high social contact with HEE relatives (Leff et al. 1985): for those patients who remained on antipsychotic medication throughout, lowering of HEE and/or degree of face to face contact was associated with a 14% relapse rate, compared with 78% for control patients on regular medication.

In chronic illness. Social stimulation leads to improvement while it occurs, but if excessive can cause relapse. Need adequate range of domestic environment with varying degrees of independence. Large custodial institutions can have adverse effects.

Psychological
Supportive attitudes in therapist, refuse to alienate or stereotype the patient, never patronise, look for meanings in psychotic symptoms, see regularly, listen, aim at recovery and assume this likely, allow maximal self-sufficiency compatible with clinical state. Interpretive therapy practised by some.

FURTHER READING

CLINICAL FEATURES

Mellor, C. S. (1982) The present status of first rank symptoms. *Brit. J. Psychiat.*, **140**, 423–424.

CAUSES

Biochemical
Mackay, A. V. P. & Crow, T. J. (1980) Positive and negative schizophrenic symptoms and the role of dopamine. *Brit. J. Psychiat.*, **137**, 379–387.

Genetic
Murray, R. M., Lewis, S. W. & Reveley, A. M. (1985) Towards an aetiological classification of schizophrenia. *Lancet*, 1023–1926.

Interactional
Hirsch, S. R. & Leff, J. P. (1975) *Abnormalities in the Parents of Schizophrenics*: Maudsley monograph No. 22. London: Oxford University Press.

TREATMENT AND OUTCOME

Drug and Therapeutics Bulletin (1987) Stopping drug treatment in schizophrenia. **25**, 31–32.

Leff, J. P. (1972) Maintenance therapy and schizophrenia. *Br. J. Hosp. Med.*, **October 8**, 377–380.

Leff, J. P., Kuipers, L., Berkowitz, R. & Sturgeon, D. (1985) A controlled trial of social intervention in the families of schizophrenic patients: two-year follow-up. *Brit. J. Psychiat.*, **146**, 594–600.

Manchanda, R. & Hirsch, S. R. (1986) Low dose maintenance. *Brit. Med. J.*, **293**, 515–516.

Kolakowska, T., Williams, A. O., Ardern, M., et al. (1985) Schizophrenia with good and poor outcome. *Brit. J. Psychiat.*, **146**, 229–246.

Vaughn, C. E. & Leff, J. P. (1976) The influence of family and social factors on the course of psychiatric illness. *Brit. J. Psychiat.*, **129**, 125–137.

Wing, J. K. (1980) *Psychiatric Rehabilitation in the 1980s*. London: Royal College of Psychiatrists.

Wing, J. K. (1985) Leading article. Relapse in schizophrenia. *Brit. Med. J.*, **291**, 1219–1220.

Watt, D. C., Katz, K. & Shepherd, M. (1983) The natural history of schizophrenia: a five-year follow-up of a representative sample of schizophrenics. *Psychol. Med.*, **13**, 663–670.

Paranoid reactions

NORMAL VARIANTS

Transient ideas of self reference may occur in normal, especially in sensitive, shy personalities.

Usually evanescent, carry no conviction and do not lead to action.

MORBID REACTIONS

More persistent with a sense of conviction, logic and coherence. May lead to action. Usually understandable in the light of situation and previous personality.

Causes

1. *Acute organic brain syndromes* (drug or alcohol withdrawal delirium, post-head injury, post-operative, myxoedema). There may be marked paranoid ideas and acutely disturbed behaviour in context of confusion, disorientation and hallucinations.
2. *Drug induced.* Amphetamine psychosis may closely resemble paranoid schizophrenia. LSD confusional hallucinatory states may contain paranoid element.
3. *Personality development.* Certain self-referring individuals may develop systems of over-valued ideas, litiginous or otherwise in absence of other symptoms which might suggest psychosis. Morbid jealousy may be a highly dangerous state with intense jealous preoccupation regarding spouse, usually concerning infidelity. Often associated with impotence in male and previous alcohol abuse.
4. *Situational.* Prolonged isolation, imprisonment, immigrant status.
   Folie à deux (Lasegue & Falret 1877) occurs in response to prolonged, more or less exclusive exposure to psychotic relative or other key individual, usually a dominant partner. Apparent delusional ideas may be identical in content with those of the psychotic individual, but more amenable to discussion and improve with separation.

59

Folie simultanée occurs when the individuals are both psychotically ill.

Group imitative disorders, especially under stress or in isolation (*folie à famille*).

5. *Physical disability*. Deafness, especially in older persons. Less common in blindness. Disfiguring lesions, especially facial, deformed limbs and when acute in onset.

6. *Complicating mental illness*. Paranoid symptoms especially common in the elderly. May complicate dementia of any kind or affective disorders, but the cardinal symptoms of these remain discernible. Late onset paranoid schizophrenia similar, and may present diagnostic difficulties.

Affective disorders

A group of illnesses of variable severity in which the central symptom is a periodic alteration of mood into either mania or depression, usually accompanied by other characteristic symptoms. (Anxiety states are considered separately under Neurotic Disorders).

CLASSIFICATION OF AFFECTIVE DISORDERS

A great deal of controversy has long existed concerning the classification of affective disorders: it exemplifies the problem of using poorly defined terms which confuse description with implied mechanism: for example psychosis, neurosis, endogenous, reactive. The situation is complicated by the need to distinguish normal day to day variation in mood from states which are significantly different for them to be recognisable as morbid.

REACTIVE (NEUROTIC) DEPRESSION. (DSMIII: MILD DEPRESSIVE DISORDER, DYSTHYMIC DISORDER)

Absence of severe depressive symptoms, such as delusions and hallucinations. Certain symptoms common, though they are relatively infrequent in psychotic affective disorder. They are: phobias, obsessional symptoms, less often hysterical symptoms. Anxiety can occur in both types of depressive disorder.

Such additional symptoms in reactive depression have led to it being called neurotic depression, with the implication that it might be qualitatively different from the more severe forms of illness and based on long standing personality problems of a neurotic kind. It is hazardous to assume this argument to be more than conjecture, and advisable to acknowledge both endogenous and reactive causal factors in every affective illness.

Whether it is called reactive, neurotic, dysthymic, or minor, this form of depressive illness is very important because it is extremely common in the general population and constitutes a significant proportion of a general practitioner's work.

AFFECTIVE PSYCHOSIS (ICD9: MANIC DEPRESSIVE PSYCHOSIS. DSMIII: MAJOR AFFECTIVE DISORDER).

In affective psychosis the mental state is severely disordered by the development of delusions and/or hallucinations, and as a result there is serious impairment of insight and judgement.

Kraepelin introduced the term manic depressive psychosis in 1921. This refers to a single disease entity, with depressive psychotic and/or manic episodes, either single or recurrent and either one or both types in the same patient. Kraepelin found that the type of symptoms did not change in successive relapses, and it was possible to return to an unimpaired level of personality function no matter how many relapses occurred (in contrast with the personality deterioration in what he called dementia praecox, later termed schizophrenia). The term manic depressive psychosis has led to major problems because it has been assumed necessarily to be 'endogenous' in nature, thereby excluding illness which appears to have developed in response to external stress, yet may have identical clinical features. Recently the terms 'unipolar' and 'bipolar' have come into favour as originally suggested by Leonhard in 1957 (see Kendell 1983).

EPIDEMIOLOGY

Female : Male 1.3–2.0 : 1.0.
Prevalence of affective psychosis as seen in general practice: 2.4–6.0/1000.
This is ten times more than referral rate to hospital.
Lifetime morbidity rates: males   4–10 per 1000 live births.
                          : females 6–28 per 1000 live births.

NATURAL HISTORY OF ILLNESS

Recurrent relapses but without deterioration of personality between episodes. 40% readmitted at least once in four years after discharge from hospital (20% more than once).

4.5% remain in hospital for one year compared with 14.5% patients suffering from schizophrenia (Norris 1955).

Episodes become more frequent and their length tends to increase with age. May be recurrent depression or mania, or any sequence of the two. Circular (bipolar) form with alternating mania and depression is uncommon, and although individual episodes of illness are shorter, they recur more frequently, and there is a higher morbid risk in first degree relatives. The bipolar and unipolar forms tend to breed true in relatives.

SYMPTOMS AND SIGNS: DEPRESSIVE PSYCHOSIS

Overt depression of mood
May be diurnal variation, worse in morning.
Vary from flatness to deep gloom.
Tearfulness (particularly significant if different from previous personality).

Disorder of thinking
Pessimism. May see no future. Loss of hope.
Suicidal ideas.
Poor concentration, mental slowness.
Delusional ideas: self-blame
                   nihilistic
                   hypochondriacal
                   paranoid.
Impatience, irritability.

Motor concomitants
Poor appetite, weight loss.
Insomnia, especially early morning waking.
Retardation, stupor.
Agitation when anxiety marked.
Multiple somatic complaints.
Constipation.
Loss of libido.

Hallucinations
Usually auditory: critical voices.

Misinterpretations
Ideas of reference, e.g. people talking about self in a critical way.
Misconstrues remarks of others.

SYMPTOMS AND SIGNS: MANIC OR HYPOMANIC PSYCHOSIS

Elevation of mood
Persistent over days or weeks.
May be punctuated by episodic depression or irritability and angry outbursts, especially when wishes are thwarted.

Disorder of thinking
Flight of ideas: impaired train of thought related to pressure of ideas and marked distractibility, impaired concentration.
   Speech may contain puns, clang associations and rhyming in context of euphoric mood.
   Delusional ideas; re financial status, personal attributes. In a minority may be paranoid.

Motor concomitants

Self-neglect, weight loss and exhaustion in severe cases.

Marked restlessness and overactivity.

Insomnia may be severe.

50% experience moderate/severe depression in first three months of convalescence.

Mania may be confused with schizophrenic excitement.

CAUSAL THEORIES

Biochemical

May be more than one underlying chemical disorder.

Biogenic amine hypothesis

Clinical depression associated with a functional deficiency of noradrenaline or serotonin at receptor sites in brain. Mania associated with excess of these agents.

Note that studies of CSF and urine are indirect: metabolite levels may reflect changes in spinal cord or even other tissues rather than the brain.

Experimental evidence based on pharmacological properties of antidepressant drugs, changes in levels of metabolites of biogenic amines in patients with affective disorders, and the effects of their precursors.

Catecholamines. MAOIs increase intraneural concentration of active amines such as noradrenaline, dopamine and serotonin. May also decrease their uptake. (Remains to be shown that MAOIs cause increased functional activity at central aminergic receptor sites.)

Tricyclic antidepressants potentiate action of endogenously released noradrenaline by blocking its re-uptake into nerve terminals.

Reserpine causes depressive-like states and depletion of catecholamines.

Indoleamines. Antidepressants have similar effects on serotonin metabolism.

Some reports suggest that CSF 5-OH-indoleacetic acid (breakdown product of serotonin) low in depression, although it remains so after recovery. Increased hepatic tryptophan pyrrolase may reduce amount of tryptophan available for serotonin synthesis.

Tryptophan potentiates the antidepressant effect of MAOIs.

Fall in levels of 5HT may occur in parallel with changes in catecholamines.

Effect of precursors. L-Tryptophan (precursor of 5HT) reported as having antidepressant effect.

Post-mortem studies of brain tissue. Unconfirmed report that 5HT levels low in brain stem of depressed patients. No change in concentration of noradrenaline or dopamine.

Change in receptor sensitivity (Ashcroft). Balance between transmitter availability and receptor sensitivity crucial. Variation in the latter may be a significant causal factor.

Endocrine

Thyroid hormones may potentiate tricyclic antidepressants by influence on receptor sensitivity (activates adenyl cyclase-cyclic AMP system which is closely related to the adrenergic receptor).

Plasma adrenocortical steroids may be raised in 50% of patients with severe depression. May be related to nonspecific stress of the illness or disordered hypothalmic function.

Some claim that the limbic system and hypothalamus are the sites of the primary pathology in the affective disorders. The dexamethasone suppression test has been used to evaluate the role of the hypothalamus-pituitary-adrenal system (HPA). In normals there is suppression of plasma cortisol for 24 hours after overnight dose of dexamethasone. Depressed individuals (20–40%) may show impaired suppression of plasma cortisol. Some authors claim that such findings are specific to 'endogenous' depression, with 'biological' symptoms and suicidal behaviour. The findings return to normal with recovery (Carroll). Other authors are more cautious (McGuffin).

The suppression test may prove useful in diagnosis (e.g. distinguishing between organic dementia and pseudodementia in the elderly) and in monitoring treatment.

Electrolyte metabolism

Electrolytes influence resting cell membrane potentials, impulse transmission and synaptic changes. Also have important role in biogenic amine release, re-uptake and storage, but no clear link as yet with causal hypotheses concerning affective disorders.

Lithium useful in therapy of affective disorders.

Intracellular sodium retention in depression, re-excretion in recovery (Gibbons). Sodium retention may occur in lithium responders.

Genetic

Familial incidence

MZ twins 68% concordance. DZ twins reared apart or together 19%. First degree relatives: 10–15%. General population 1–2%.

Unipolar and bipolar forms tend to breed true.

No excess of schizophrenia among relatives of depressive patients.

Possible genetic mechanisms
Single dominant autosomal gene. Incomplete penetrance because not all patients have affected parent, not all MZ twins concordant, rate less than 50% in sibs and children of patients.

Polygenic. This might explain continuum of severity of affective illnesses in general population.

Some degree of X-linkage. Greater than chance association with X linked marker traits, e.g. Xg blood system, dentan and protan colour blindness, certain HLA antigens.

Psychological

Psychoanalytic
Loss of love object. Libido withdrawn and invested in the ego which becomes identified with the lost object and subjected to sadistic impulses of the original ambivalent libidinous cathexis.

Early loss
Severe depression associated with loss of parent before age of 20. Severely depressed patients also show increased incidence of loss of parent through death during the 20 years preceding admission — applies only to patients under 40 years (Birtchnell).

Premorbid personality
Cyclothymia (tendency to mood swings) more common. Possibly also anxiety and obsessional features predispose.

Adaptation model
Depressive symptoms serve a protective purpose by reducing responsiveness (due to habituation through chronic frustration and lack of reinforcement). Seligman: learned helplessness.

Cognitive theory of depression (Beck)
This postulates depressive syndrome as a process of 'cognitive shift' involving three areas of cognitive dysfunction. Predisposing habitual patterns of thinking. These are:
negative cognitive triad involving pervading themes related to the self, the world and the future;
logical system errors leading to erroneous conclusions and attitudes (arbitrary inference, selective abstraction, personalisation, overgeneralisation, magnification, minimisation);
idiosyncratic schemes which act as enduring cognitive templates which screen, code, categorise and evaluate information.

'Reactive' vs 'Endogenous' depression

Based on whether the symptoms occur independently of environmental causes (endogenous) or appear to be a response to external stressors (reactive). There has also been a tendency to equate 'endogenous' with 'psychotic' and 'reactive' with 'neurotic'. In practice, this has been extremely unreliable. Clinical techniques for deciding degree of reactivity are rudimentary. Confusion has also occurred in use of the term 'psychotic', some interpreting it strictly to mean the presence of delusions, and/or hallucination, others using it when 'biological' symptoms (weight loss, impaired libido, sleep disturbance) are significant. The term 'neurotic' too is used loosely, either in a descriptive way or to imply underlying mechanisms based on repressed anxiety.

It has been fashionable to distinguish separate endogenous and reactive syndromes: the clinical features of these are listed below but they are unreliable. Some have suggested that neurotic depression is a mild form of affective disorder which has no qualitative difference from the others. It is best to approach each illness episode as due to a combination of both endogenous and reactive causal factors.

'Reactive' v 'endogenous' depression

Neurotic (reactive)
Reactivity of depression
Rapid mood changes
Psychological precipitation
Hysterical + anxiety symptoms
Previous symptoms:
  hysterical
  anxiety
  obsessional
  bodily preoccupation
  mood variation
Childhood neurotic traits
Irritability
Hypochondriacal attitude
Demonstrative suicidal attempt
Suicidal feelings

Poor response to
antidepressants, ECT

Psychotic (endogenous)
Disturbance of food intake,
weight
Delusions:
  guilt
  unworthiness
  bodily change
  persecution
Ideas of reference
Suspiciousness
Perplexity
Severe insomnia
Apathy
Agitation
Social withdrawal
Speech: abnormal rate or
quantity
Auditory hallucinations
Family history of affective
psychosis
Good response to
antidepressants, ECT

Studies from Newcastle described a bimodal distribution of symptoms, suggesting two distinct clinical entities. Kendell suggests this finding might be an artefact due to patient selection and 'halo' effects: when consecutive patients rated, distribution is unimodal. The two syndromes may be at opposite ends of depressive continuum, most patients fall somewhere between, having a mixture of both kinds of symptom.

Linear relation between score on neurotic/psychotic scale and response to ECT. Multiple causation compatible with this.

Environmental: life event studies
Interpretation difficult. Association may be coincidental, non-specific or due to spurious reconstruction either as part of random search for causes, or due to distortion of attitudes produced by illness itself.

Adverse life events increased in frequency in all types of affective disorders: includes hypomania (20% preceded by adverse life event — Leff). Paykel found 6-fold increase in risk of developing depression in 6 months following markedly threatening life events.

Social: the Brown and Harris study
Depressed women in urban community. Interviewed 114 psychiatric patients and 458 women in random community sample. Assessed situational and life-event causal factors: emphasis placed not merely on change but also its meaning for the individual. Formulated causal theory of depression which accords central importance to social factors. Life events relevant only if perceived as long-term threat. In this research the significant personal meaning of a life event is evaluated contextually by the investigator, not in terms of the patient's viewpoint.

Provoking factors
Either severe event or major life difficulty. 'Severe event' defined as experience of loss or disappointment concerning a person, object, role or idea (e.g. real or threatened separation from key figure, major material loss, general disappointment, miscellaneous crises such as work redundancy). 'Major life difficulties' were those of at least 2 years duration (excluding problems of health).

15% of women were considered to have suffered from affective disorder in the 3 months before interview. 8% were 'onset cases' in

which depression had commenced at some time in the pre
year.

83% of onset cases had experienced severe event or majo
difficulty.

61% of cases ⎫ had experienced at least one severe
19% of non cases ⎬ event in the preceding nine months
29% of patients did not have provoking factors

Provoking factors important in both psychotic and neurotic depression. Only 20% of provoking factors followed by depression, the development of which requires the presence of vulnerability factors.

Vulnerability factors
These become causal only in the presence of provoking agent.
They do not in themselves lead to depression.
They are: — absence of confiding relationship
— lack of mother (not father) before age 11 years
— lack of employment outside home
— looking after young children (3 or more children under 14 years of age)
They act by lowering self esteem, thereby impairing ability to cope with provoking factors and leading to the central depressive triad in which the self seems worthless, the future hopeless and the world meaningless. They are more common in working-class women, and explain why these are four times more likely than middle-class women to develop depressive disorder in face of provoking agent. The class difference is restricted to women with children. Less important cause of social class difference was increased experience of severe life events and major life difficulties in working-class women.

Symptom formation factors
These are related to the overall severity of depression.
They are — past loss
— age over 40 years
— previous episode
The presence of all three symptom formation factors strongly related to absence of provoking agent.
Psychotic depression related to loss by death
Neurotic depression related to loss by separation

MIXED AFFECTIVE STATES

Depressive and manic symptoms may occur in the patient during one and the same illness episode, or follow each other in rapid sequence.

INVOLUTIONAL MELANCHOLIA

Not a distinct entity: depression in elderly does not differ in any fundamental way from that in younger patients either symptomatically or genetically. Hypochondriacal delusions probably due to pathoplastic effects of age. Probably of no value.

DEPRESSION IN CHILDHOOD

Approximately 15–20% of children referred for psychiatric help, 1.4% of 10-year-olds, 4% of 14-year-olds have depressive disorder. Girls more vulnerable than boys, more common in preschool children and adolescents than in primary school children. Commonly co-exists with other syndromes such as conduct disorder, hyperkinesis.

DIFFERENTIAL DIAGNOSIS OF DEPRESSIVE ILLNESS

1. Chronic organic brain disorder (dementia): may be retarded and slow. Look for defect in memory and orientation (conversely, depressive illness may mimic organic brain disorder when poor concentration and retardation cause difficulty in eliciting cognitive function).
2. Schizophrenia. In early stages before florid symptoms become evident.
3. Excessive medication: night sedation, especially in elderly, phenobarbitone in epileptics.
4. Drug abuse: self-neglect, withdrawal from amphetamine.
5. Certain therapeutic drugs: reserpine, methyldopa, diuretics, sympathetic blockers.
6. Endocrine disorders: hypothyroidism, hypopituitarism.
7. Neurotic disorders: anxiety, phobic, obsessional. In all these an underlying depressive illness must be searched for carefully.
8. Depressive personality: in this case the individual has a disability of long standing and it is unwise to embark on intensive physical therapy.

DIFFERENTIAL DIAGNOSIS OF HYPOMANIA OR MANIA

1. Schizophrenia may cause excitement and overactivity. Differentiation can be difficult because mania may lead to delusions and hallucinations resembling those found in schizophrenia.

2. Organic brain disorder: especially frontal lobe lesions which may cause disinhibition.
3. Drug abuse: LSD, amphetamines.
4. Epilepsy: post-ictal excitement.

TREATMENT OF DEPRESSIVE ILLNESS

PSYCHOTHERAPY

Supportive relationship can be very beneficial. See regularly. Avoid facile reassurance although maintain an optimistic approach. Investigate physical symptoms only on their intrinsic merit, not merely to reassure. Dissuade from major changes in life, e.g. resignation from job when depressed or hypomanic. Hospital admission if: persistent disabling affective symptoms, significant risk of suicide, poor social support or family intolerance hinder recovery. Use interpretive psychotherapy after affective symptoms resolved: aim to clarify precipitating factors and facilitate adjustment to them, involve 'key other' persons in therapy where possible. Early causal factors may also be discussed in more prolonged formal therapy.

Cognitive therapy

An active directive time-limited structured approach. May be used in a variety of disorders. In the treatment of depression it aims to help the patient to
— develop a more positive attitude
— stop unjustified thoughts which negate this view
— adopt thoughts that uphold it.
    Appeal to facts of day to day behaviour (use of diary) in order to disprove false ideas.
    Useful in mild to moderate depression, particularly as adjunct to physical methods of treatment, or alone when these are inappropriate.

DRUGS

Pharmacology of antidepressant drugs

Tricyclics: tertiary amines (e.g. amitriptyline, imipramine, clomipramine, trimipramine, doxepin, dibenzepin). Other drugs such as chlorpromazine may compete with enzymic oxidation in liver, with resulting slower breakdown.
    Adjustment of dose relatively easy because response increases with dose which can be pushed to limit of tolerance.
Tricyclics: secondary amines (e.g. nortriptyline, desimipramine, protriptyline): effectiveness may be reduced in high doses.
    All tricyclic antidepressants reduce the uptake of hypertensive agents into adrenergic neurones and render them ineffective. Avoid

combining the two. Their atropine-like action may cause serious synergism with other drugs and lead to glaucoma, ileus, urinary retention.

Overdose may cause coma, convulsions, hypertension, cardiac dysrhythmias, and hallucinations during recovery.

Monoamine oxidase inhibitors (MAOIs): monoamine oxidase enzyme block intestinal absorption of tyramine which is an indirect sympathomimetic amine: does not act on adrenergic receptors but provokes release of catecholamines which cause hypertension with or without hyperpyrexia.

MAOIs block the intestinal protective mechanism, and foods containing sufficient tyramine may cause dangerous reactions.

Foods to be avoided: mature cheeses, pickled herrings, yeast, meat extracts (Marmite, Bovril), Chianti, beer, sherry, game, badly stored meat, any protein food that is not fresh, banana skins, broad bean pods (dopa). Treatment cards should be carried (prepared by BMA and Pharmaceutical Society, and available at pharmacies).

MAOIs interact with:

a. Tyramine-like drugs, which include amphetamine, mephentermine and other pressors, ephedrine, phenylephrine and other nasal decongestants, phenylpropanolamine (proprietary cough and cold cures), fenfluramine, phenmetrazine, chlorphentermine, and other amphetamine-like anti-obesity agents, levodopa.
b. Tricyclic antidepressants, especially when MAOIs have been commenced first. Must be free from MAOIs *as well as* tricyclic drugs for 1 week before starting combined therapy. If one is discontinued, it may not be safe to restart. Use of combined therapy is best left to specialist centres.
c. Other MAOIs. Always leave an interval of time before changing from one to another.
d. Miscellaneous. Pethidine, α-methyl dopa, reserpine, may potentiate hypoglycaemic drugs, prolong action of barbiturates, chloral hydrate and alcohol.

Metabolism of MAOIs: in 46% rapid acetylation occurs with poor response. Need flexible dosage programme.

Tryptophane may potentiate antidepressant effect of MAOIs.

Mortality of therapy with antidepressant drugs: annual deaths (per 10^6 prescription): amitriptyline 2.3, phenelzine 17.2.

Tricyclics may predispose to sudden death under stress, the risk increased $\times$ 8 with exercise in cold. Cardiac dysrhythmias may complicate overdose.

N.B. 15% of individuals with affective psychosis eventually die through suicide.

DRUG MANAGEMENT OF DEPRESSION

(See Shaw)

Tricyclic drugs. Sufficient tertiary amine type drug to cause mild side effects for 4 weeks, then 7–10 days at slightly lower dose. First choice when patient mildly or moderately ill in absence of heart disease (amitriptyline 75 mg, single dose at night, increasing to 150 mg after 4 days). If ineffective in 28 days, no point in continuing.

If using secondary amine type drug and no response, reduce dose slightly in case optimal dose is low.

Newer antidepressants. Flupenthixol: low toxicity. Useful in elderly; depot decanoate available.

Tetracyclics: (mianserin, maprotiline).

MAOIs. Not all clinicians accept their use as justifiable. Patients should be able to exercise dietary discretion and avoid impulsive overdoses. Contraindicated when arteriosclerosis or liver disease present.

Phenelzine: dose difficult to judge because of variable rate of acetylation.

Isocarboxazid: weak but useful in older patients, 20–30 mg per day.

Tranylcypromine: more reliable. Stimulant. 20 mg mane, 10 mg midday, for 3 weeks. Usually effective with 3 weeks' treatment at doses causing mild side effects such as postural hypotension. Maximum dose 60 mg daily.

Lithium carbonate. Valuable in reducing the relapse rate of bipolar disorders, whether for manic or depressive episodes. This renders lithium carbonate particularly useful in such patients because tricyclic drugs and ECT are liable to precipitate manic relapse. Evidence is less convincing in unipolar depressive disorders, and the less toxic antidepressant drugs are preferred.

ECT IN DEPRESSION

First choice therapy in moderate/severe depression when suicidal risk serious and/or little response to drug therapy. May need 3–4 unilateral treatments in first week if severe. Maximum of 12 applications in one course.

TREATMENT OF MANIA

PSYCHOTHERAPY

As in depression.

DRUGS

(See also pp. 154–157)

Haloperidol: drug of first choice. 10–30 mg i.m. Monitor blood pressure — should not fall below 100 mgHg systolic. Repeat at 1–1½ h intervals until mania subsides: may need 40–100 mg per day initially. Switch to oral therapy as soon as possible (oral dose = 2 × i.m. dose).

Lithium carbonate: commence at same time as haloperidol, delay of 10 days before it acts. 0.8–1.0 mEq./L. Dose 1000–1200 mg per day. Check serum level every 5 days initially.

Phenothiazines: if chlorpromazine used, give test dose 10 mg i.m. and monitor for hypotension. 50–75 mg i.m. every 30–45 minutes until improvement occurs. Maximum 200 mg in 3 h. Only give antiparkinsonian drugs if needed.

TREATMENT OF RECURRENT AFFECTIVE ILLNESS

Tricyclic antidepressants maintained for 6 months after episode of depression reduce risk of relapse to about 50% (Mindham et al.). Not effective in mania or bipolar illnesses.

If maintenance lithium proposed: check renal, cardiac functions and make sure not pregnant or planning to be. Stop lithium if become pregnant.

Caution if intercurrent disease or currently taking diuretics. Check blood levels exactly 12 hours after last dose.

Side effects of lithium: nausea, loose stools, vomiting, diarrhoea, tremor of hands (coarse tremor may herald serious toxicity), polyuria, polydipsia, weight gain, oedema, sluggishness, sleepiness, vertigo, dysarthria. Occasionally hypothyroid goitre (treat with 0.1–0.2 mg thyroxin daily, but may have to stop lithium). May be fatal coma in severe overdosage. Slow excretion of drug makes treatment of overdose difficult.

FURTHER READING

Beck, A. T., Rush, B. F. & Emery, G. (1979) *Cognitive therapy of depression.* New York: Guildford Press.

Birtchnell, J. (1970) Depression in relation to early and recent parental death. *Brit. J. Psychiat.,* **116**, 229–306.

Black, D. (1987) Leading article. Depression in children. *Brit. Med. J.,* **294**, 462–463.

Brown, G. W. et al. (1977) Depression and loss. *Brit. J. Psychiat.,* **130**, 1–18.

Brown, G. W. & Harris, T. (1978) *Social origins of depression.* London: Tavistock.

Brown, G. W., Bifulco, A. & Harris, T. O. (1987) Life events, vulnerability and onset of depression. *Brit. J. Psychiat.,* **150**, 30–43.

Carroll, B. J. (1982) The dexamethasone suppression test for melancholia. *Brit. J. Psychiat.,* **140**, 292–304.

Kendell, R. E. (1968) *The Classification of Depressive Illness.*

Kendell, R. E. (1983) In *Companion to Psychiatric Studies*, 3rd Edn. Ed. Kendell, R. E. & Zeally, A. K. Edinburgh: Churchill Livingstone. Maudsley Monograph No. 18. London: Oxford University Press.

McGuffin, P. (1984) Editorial. Biological markers and psychosis. *Psychol. Med.*, **14**, 255–258.

Mindham, R. H. S. & Shepherd, M. (1973) An evaluation of continuation therapy with tricyclic antidepressants in depressive illness. *Psychol. Med.*, **3**, 5–17.

Paykel, E. S. (1983) *Handbook of Affective Disorders*. Ed. Paykel, E. S. Edinburgh: Churchill Livingstone.

Shaw, D. M. (1973) Biochemical basis of affective disorders. *Brit. J. Hosp. Med.*, Nov. 1973, 609–616.

Shaw, D. M. (1977) The practical management of affective disorders. *Brit. J. Psychiat.*, **130**, 430–451.

BEREAVEMENT REACTIONS

Typical (uncomplicated) grief

Initial short period of emotional 'numbness'.

Episodic emotional distress, becoming less severe in 1–2 months.

Off work for short periods (2 weeks). No psychiatric consultation needed.

Severity and type of distress may vary even within the same individual from one episode of bereavement to another, depending on the precise nature of the loss in each instance. Disturbing sense of loss may last many months.

Preoccupation with memories of the deceased
May be clear visual imagery.
Idealise the dead person.

Perceptual disturbances
Misinterpret sounds as due to the deceased.
Misidentify other persons as being the deceased.
Sense of presence.
Visual hallucinations, occasional auditory.

Mental distress
Depression, withdrawal, guilt (suicidal ideas 11%).
Episodic yearning, anxiety.

Physical symptoms
Headaches, vomiting, anorexia, chest pains, dyspnoea, joint pains (may resemble symptoms in dead person's final illness).

Behavioural changes
Social withdrawal, restlessness. Conduct aimed at keeping memory alive.
Preservation of possessions (mummification).

Hostility
Anger at those responsible for care of the deceased during terminal illness.
Loss of compassion for others.
Anger at being abandoned.

Increased mortality risk
4.76% first degree relatives in first year, 0.86% controls (Rees & Lutkins.)
Suicide increased $\times$ 2.5 in first year. Risk greatest in widowers. 40% increase in death from coronary thrombosis, cancer, respiratory infections.

Long term effects
Childhood bereavement may predispose to psychiatric illness in adulthood, particularly depression. Increased risk of alcoholism in men. Chronic poor physical health (43%).

Atypical (complicated) grief
May take various forms.

Absence of grief.
Excessively delayed (related to phobic avoidance, extreme guilt, anger). Parkes and Weiss have recently identified two major types of delayed grief reaction:
— The unexpected grief syndrome: follows unexpected major loss. Disbelief may delay full reaction, but anxiety is high. Continued sense of obligation and presence delays resolution.
— The ambivalent grief syndrome: immediate sense of relief gives way to intense pining, sometimes self punitive behaviour.
Chronic grief. In this form the grief is expressed in full from the outset but excessively prolonged. Often anger over care of the deceased. More severe (suicide attempts, excessive guilt, severe depression, anger, intense social withdrawal).
   Psychosomatic symptoms may predominate (e.g. hypertension, diabetes, duodenal ulcer, asthma, ulcerative colitis). Recent reports suggest suppression of immune response (lymphocyte T function).
   Certain symptoms particularly common: difficulty in accepting the loss (refusal), marked hostility to others, identification with personality traits and symptoms of deceased, excessive idealisation, recurrent nightmares, avoidance of memories, objects or places associated with deceased, anniversary reactions, panic attacks.

Factors associated with increased risk (Parkes 1985)

Type of death:
  (i)   cause for blame on survivor
  (ii) sudden or unexpected
  (iii) painful, horrifying, mismanaged.

The relationship:
  (i) Dependent or symbiotic
  (ii) Ambivalent
  (iii) Spouse dies (leaving widower)
  (iv) Child or young adult under 20 years dies
  (v) Parent dies leaving children aged 5 years or less, or 10–15 years
  (vi) Parent dies leaving older, unmarried adult.

The survivor:
  (i) Grief-prone (dependent)
  (ii) Over-anxious with low self esteem
  (iii) Previous mental illness
  (iv) Excessively angry
  (v) Very self reproachful
  (vi) Physically disabled
  (vii) Previous unresolved losses
  (viii) Unable to express feelings.

Social circumstances:
  (i) Family absent or unsupportive
  (ii) Detached from traditional support systems for example immigrants
  (iii) Unemployed
  (iv) Dependent children
  (v) Low socio-economic status.

Treatment

About 1 in 3 reactions to major losses require some kind of specialised help.

Helping the work of grieving: realisation, making real the loss, disengagement. Formal ritual aspects of mourning helpful. Western society tends to lack traditional ritual and belief systems which support the bereaved. In early stages individual or family support at home best. Aim to facilitate expression of grief, reassure about significance of physical and psychological symptoms. Ensure time and space to grieve, monitor risks, for example suicide. Psychiatrists can play useful role in supporting befrienders and counsellors (Cruse).

Helping strategies. Listen, encourage to express feelings (especially after the funeral is over). Psychotropic drugs when symptoms severe. Beware of validation of sick role, and suppression of the normal physiological mechanisms of grief with a risk of prolonging the process. Self help groups (beware they do not encourage perpetuation of grief). Exploit social 'bridges' at turning point in grief. Important to recognise and deal with defence mechanisms such as denial, projection, idealisation.

Morbid grief may be resistant to treatment. When avoidance behaviour predominates, a 'forced mourning' procedure is often effective (Lieberman 1978, Mawson et al. 1981).

Forced mourning ineffective, perhaps harmful, in those who have inadequate family support and significant social problems.

Other relatives may share morbid grief and may also be included in forced mourning procedure.

Later stages of helping process should focus increasingly on establishing new life style and bridges: group counselling helpful. In chronic grief it may be important to aim at giving permission for grief to end, rather than continue as a duty and enduring obligation.

FURTHER READING

Brown, G. W. et al. (1977) Depression and loss. *Brit. J. Psychiat.*, **130**, 1–18.

Granville-Grossman, K. (1971) In *Recent Advances in Clinical Psychiatry-1*. pp. 180–191. Edinburgh: Churchill Livingstone.

Lieberman, S. (1978) Nineteen cases of morbid grief. *Brit. J. Psychiat.*, **132**, 159–163.

Mawson, D., Marks, I.M., Ramm, L. & Stern, R. S. (1981) Guided mourning for morbid grief: a controlled study. *Brit. J. Psychiat.*, **138**, 185–193.

Parkes, C. M. (1972) *Bereavement: Studies of Grief in Adult Life*. London: Tavistock.

Parkes, C. M. (1985) Review article. Bereavement. *Brit. J. Psychiat.*, **146**, 11–17.

Rees, W. D. & Lutkins, S. G. (1967) Mortality of bereavement. *Brit. Med. J.*, **4**, 13–16.

Worden, W. (1982) *Grief Counselling and Grief Therapy*. London: Tavistock.

The neuroses

A. HYSTERIA

A psychological reaction at an unconscious level and related to chronic unresolved internal conflict or acute external stress.

May show belle indifference: lack of anxiety and concern over disability caused by hysterical symptoms.

HISTORICAL BACKGROUND

For many centuries hysteria was regarded as a strange disease entity confined to women, originating in the uterus and related to frustrated sexual drive.

In the 19th century there was a re-awakening of scientific interest in it. The study of hysteria figured prominently in the early development of psychodynamic theories.

Mesmer: animal magnetism transferrable between individuals. Rapport important.

Briquet (1859): first systematic study. Emphasised preponderance in females, in lower social class, and the causal importance of heredity as well as violent emotional upset.

Charcot (1870): At the Salpetrière, Paris. Over-emphasised neurological disease entity approach: arbitrary definitions. Peculiar atmosphere of mental contagion and suggestibility surrounded his practice, when symptoms were produced on demand in theatrical setting. La Grande Hysterie. Distinguished hysterical from true fits. Hypnotism eventually regarded as a feature of hysteria.

Babinski (1901): led reaction against Charcot. Maintained hysteria merely the end result of suggestion.

P. Janet (1880s): Emphasised causal importance of repression of painful ideas into unconscious.

Freud (1886): Began work on hysteria.

CLINICAL FEATURES

Symptoms of two types

a. Conversion
Psychogenic disorder of bodily function greater than normal psychosomatic interaction. May take form of paralysis, ataxia, tremor, blindness, deafness, pseudo epilepsy, syncope. Pain may be the most common. May include a variety of psychological symptoms e.g. hallucinations, depression.

Conversion symptoms can be distinguished from those due to organic disease by:
1. variability
2. lack of objective evidence of organic disease
3. atypicality (e.g. disturbance of sensory loss, type of ataxia)
4. inconsistency (apparently paralysed muscles may show normal power when acting as synergists, or weakness may be due to contraction of antagonists)
5. loss of function reflects patient's concept of disability rather than neuro-anatomical principles.

b. Dissociation
Psychogenic disorders involving impairment of personal awareness. May take the form of amnesia, clouding, apparent disorientation, with or without fugue state, alternate personality.

Dissociative amnesia often global, involving total recall in absence of evidence of organic brain disorder but with retention of registration, recall for immediate past, and skills in reading, writing and arithmetic. May selectively involve memory loss for emotionally upsetting events.

Secondary gain
This is frequently discernible, but scrupulous clinical evaluation and judgement needed in view of the gross unreliability of this concept.

May complicate true organic disease
Organic disease may present with symptoms which are partly or completely due to hysterical mechanisms.

Temporal lobe epilepsy particularly liable to precipitate hysterical symptoms.

Of 85 patients with 'hysteria' followed up 9 years later, 66% were found to have developed florid organic disease: this had not been detected clinically when hysteria diagnosed at first, but had probably played a part in leading to initial symptoms (Slater).

'Hysterical' syndromes in which organic causes likely (Merskey)
Paroxysmal hemicrania.
Thoracic outlet syndrome.
Globus hystericus (globus pharyngis). 307 patient series of
Malcolmson, 30% of whom had local physical lesions which
probably had a causal role. They included thyroid goitre, enlarged
lymph nodes, postcricoid web, cervical spinal osteophytes. Forty-
nine per cent of patients had gastrointestinal disorder such as hiatus
hernia, duodenal ulcer.
Facial dyskinesia, torticollis. The former can be precipitated by
levodopa and phenothiazines.
Note that secondary symptoms of anger, frustration when multiple
medical referrals seem fruitless, should not be confused with
primary causal factors.

Symptom groupings (Reed)
113 patients: detailed clinical analysis and follow up mean 11.7
years.
A. 13% conversion/dissociative only. No other symptoms
   developed. Often single illness.
B. 33% conversion/dissociative with affective symptoms
   (depression, anxiety, preceded or followed original episode).
C. 28% affective symptoms only. More aptly termed histrionic
   behaviour.
D. 21% other syndromes present (e.g. schizophrenia, agoraphobia).
E. 5% uncertain diagnosis.
   Concludes: Group A represents discrete syndrome of pure
'hysteria' characterised by conversion/dissociation, belle
indifference and secondary gain in absence of other symptoms.

Clinical syndromes (Merskey)
A. Single motor, sensory or dissociative symptoms, sometimes
   including pain.
B. Polysymptomatic e.g. hypochondriasis and *Briquet's* syndrome.
C. Elaboration of organic complaint.
D. Self induced illness or self damage in abnormal personality.
E. Psychotic or pseudo psychotic disorders (Ganser Syndrome,
   hysterical psychosis).
F. Hysterical personality.
G. Culturally sanctioned: endemic or epidemic.

Munchausen syndrome
Recurrent presentation to hospitals, simulated organic disease, may
lead to unnecessary major medical or surgical intervention. Some
cases follow episodes of true organic disease. Seek relief in sick role.
Level of conscious awareness of underlying motives uncertain.
Formulation mainly in terms of malingering, inadequate.

Alternative personalities. Based on dissociative mechanisms: the individual may appear to switch between two different personalities of disparate behaviour and attitudes.

AETIOLOGY
Slater suggests there is no such entity as hysteria, merely hysterical symptoms which may complicate other conditions.

Reed distinguishes a pure entity of 'hysteria' and provided it is strictly defined, argues for its retention.

Psychoanalytic theory
Repressed anxiety due to instinctual impulses lead to hysterical symptoms which often have symbolic meaning and secondary gain. Radical resolution of conflict is avoided. In some cases this may be sexual: the Oedipus complex (the nuclear process in the neurosis) is seen as particularly relevant to hysteria, remaining at the phallic phase of sexual development (Fenichel). Phobic anxiety seen as form of anxiety hysteria, repressed anxiety, displaced on to neutral object or situation.

Genetic
Increased incidence of hysteria in relatives of hysterics, but they also show a similar increase in variety of other conditions (Ljungberg). No significant twin concordance.

Suggestion and shared anxiety
Outbreaks of mass hysteria in certain communities. Charcot produced hysterical symptoms by strong suggestion and saw hysteria as disease entity.

Personality
In 40% of cases of hysteria, preceding 'hysterical' traits: dependent, manipulative, egocentric, attention seeking, histrionic, labile and superficial emotionality.

Beware of pejorative misuse of these terms. Chodoff urges that we discard the concept of hysterical personality: dubious validity and uncertain relationships to hysteria.

Patients with hysterical pain have characteristic high MMPI scores for hypochondriasis and hysteria, low for depression (the V triad).

Sick role
Seek this through learnt behaviour in face of intolerable life difficulties, conflict or physical disease. Variable degree of conscious awareness of mechanism for symptoms, and delineation from malingering often highly arbitrary.

Kendell (1974) proposed that hysteria is a reaction to emotional stress/conflict in response to variety of factors: illness rewarding situations, female gender, youth, inferior social status, immigrant status, low intelligence, hysterical or passive-dependent immature personality, suggestibility, difficulty in overt expression of feelings, tendency to dissociate and use denial mechanisms in coping with stress. The resulting hysterical syndrome mimics organic disease, and consequent sick role leads to relief from precipitating stress or conflict. Fenton (1986) suggests that underlying organic brain disease may also predispose to the development of hysterical symptoms.

Compensation neurosis
More common in less severe injuries and in those involving compensation. Improvement when claim is settled. May be related to poor verbal fluency, more common in social classes IV and V and in poorly educated, particularly recent immigrants.

Tarsh and Royston: 35 claimants with accident neurosis followed up 1–7 years after claim settled. Few recovered and improvements appeared unrelated to time when compensation settled. Overprotective relatives may play important perpetuating role.

TREATMENT

Rapid spontaneous recovery of acute reactions when removed from causative stress. Communication model often useful: concentrates on the meaning of the disability conveyed to others or in terms of internal conflict. Emphasise psychotherapy when reaction is based on long-standing emotional conflict. Avoid undue preoccupation with physical symptoms: investigate them only as far as medically indicated not merely as a method of reassurance. Minimise advantages of sick role.

Taylor: analysis of the predicament which has proved intolerable but unresolvable: negotiation with the allies (persons who foster its perpetuation): selection of a dignified alternative by a figure powerful enough to alter firmly rooted beliefs.

PROGNOSIS

Depends on the associated condition, environmental problems and resilience of personality or causative problems.
Good: Acute onset, nature of conflict clear, resolvable social factors or related to drug intoxication.
Poor: Related to intractible personality or situational problems, patient remains hostile and unwilling to cooperate in treatment.

Ljungberg: 43% males, 35% females had residual symptoms after 1 year.

Lewis: 40% well and working 5 years later (Maudsley Hospital inpatients).

Carter: 70% well 4–6 years later (acute conversion reaction).

FURTHER READING

SYMPTOMS

Merskey, H. (1978) Brit. J. Hosp. Med., 19, 305–310.

DIAGNOSIS

Chodoff, P. (1974) Am. J. Psychiat., 131, 1073–1078.
Fenton, G. W. (1986) Epilepsy and hysteria. Brit. J. Psychiat., 149, 28–37.
Guze, S. B., Gloninger, C. R., Martin, R. L. & Clayton, P. J. (1986) A follow-up and family study of Briquet's syndrome. Brit. J. Psychiat., 149, 17–23.
Kendell, R. E. Medicine (1972–1974 Series) 1780–1783.
Mayou, R. (1984) Sick role, illness behaviour and coping. Brit. J. Psychiat., 144, 320–322.
Merskey, H. (1986) The importance of hysteria. Brit. J. Psychiat., 149, 23–27.
Reed, J. L. (1975) Psychological Medicine, 5, 13–17.
Reed, J. L. (1978) Compensation neurosis and Munchausen syndrome. Brit. J. Hosp. Med., 19, 314–325.
Slater, E. (1965) Brit. Med. J., 1, 1395–1399.
Tarsh, M. J. & Royston, C. (1985) A follow-up study of accident neurosis. Brit. J. Psychiat., 146, 18–25.
Taylor, D. C. (1986) Hysteria, play acting and courage. Brit. J. Psychiat., 149, 37–41.

THE GANSER SYNDROME

The syndrome
Ganser 1897 described syndrome in 3 prisoners as an 'Unusual Hysterical Confusional State':

Disordered consciousness with subsequent amnesia.

Hallucinations.

Sensory changes of hysterical type.

Vorbiereden (approximate and absurd answers).

Abrupt termination.

Rare to see complete syndrome but Ganser-type symptoms more common (Scott, Whitlock).

Not necessarily restricted to prison populations.

Uncertain whether primarily hysterical, organic confusion or schizophrenic reaction.

Verbal responses resemble early stage of dysphasia.

Difficult to define concept of 'approximate' answers: may be more in nature of random responses (some correct, others absurd).

May complicate variety of other illnesses — organic brain disease or psychotic states. Clouding of consciousness essential, otherwise suspect hysterical pseudo-dementia, malingering or buffoonery type schizophrenia.

FURTHER READING

Scott, P. D. (1965) *Brit. J. Criminology*, **5**, 127–134.
Whitlock, F. A. (1965) *Brit. J. Psychiat.*, **113**, 12–29.

B. OBSESSIVE COMPULSIVE STATES

ICD9 DEFINITION

The outstanding symptom is feeling of subjective compulsion — which must be resisted — to carry out some action, to dwell on an idea, to recall an experience, or to ruminate on an abstract topic. The symptoms are perceived by the patient to be inappropriate or nonsensical, and recognised as alien to the personality but coming from within the self. Obsessional actions may be quasi-ritualistic, designed to relieve anxiety, e.g. hand washing. Attempts at avoidance may lead to intense anxiety.

HISTORY

Janet emphasised irresolute hesitant attitudes (*Folie du doute*) and introduced concept of a single neurosis encompassing variety of phenomena. Coined term 'psychasthenia': a failure of will and attention, pathological diminution of mental energy.

Epidemiology

68% onset before 25 years of age. Average age onset 22.5 years (SD 12.1 years). One year prevalence rates 0.1–2.3/1000.
   Morbid risk decreases with increasing age.
   More common in females.

CLINICAL FEATURES

Abnormal mental content (idea, image, impulse or movement) having a subjective sense of compulsion over-riding an internal resistance. Recognised by the patient on quiet reflection as being abnormal and irrational. Obsessional ideas (ruminations) are subjective mental events. Compulsive rituals abnormal and irrational, involve motor movement. Resistance is associated with increased anxiety. Repetition an important feature, associated only with transient anxiety reduction.

Distinguish from delusional ideas which may also be repetitive and preoccupying, but are regarded by the patient as logical and true.

Affective symptoms such as phobias are only strictly obsessional if they possess all the diagnostic criteria, e.g. fear associated with obsessional compulsive symptoms.

Content often concerned with fear of harming, or contaminating others. Cleaning behaviour and avoidance of fearful stimuli the most common compulsive features. Primary ideas may lead to secondary rituals, e.g. washing which then becomes obsessional in quality. Criminal obsessional acts rare but in small minority self control may be overwhelmed, especially when previous personality shows recurrent aggressive behaviour, alcohol abuse is present, or depression is marked. Obsessional fears of harming baby may develop in puerperium: need to distinguish from depressive or other psychosis where risk of harming self and/or baby is severe.

DIFFERENTIAL DIAGNOSIS

Anxiety or phobic neurosis, depressive illness, schizophrenia, organic cerebral disorders. Careful attention to clinical features and phenomenology required. Secondary affective symptoms also common.

AETIOLOGY

Need to distinguish childhood ritualistic play behaviour which is common and normal.

Psychological theory
Defect in arousal system: major defensive reaction precipitated by minor stimuli. Leads to placatory activity which serves as a failure defence in the control of unpleasant internal states (Beech).

Anankastic personality
Carries increased risk: excessive preoccupation with orderliness, cleanliness, vacillating, conscientious, checking, anxiety prone, rigid.

Complicating other illness
Depressive illness (found in 20%): close relation with depression, both have periodic course
Anorexia nervosa (20%)
Schizophrenia
Early dementia
Post-encephalitis lethargica (uncertain whether strictly obsessional/compulsive).

Psychoanalytic theory
Defensive regression to anal sadistic phase of development leading to ambivalence, magical thinking, fear of effects of obsessional thoughts, increase in number of taboo objects with punitive superego. Due to conflict at oedipal genital stage of libidinal development.
Defence mechanisms against unconscious aggressive impulses.

Secondary gain
May be an initiating or perpetuating factor.

TREATMENT
Ensure that depressive symptoms are effectively treated.

Drugs
Do not use electively but may be necessary to control severe affective disturbance. Anafranil useful, but therapeutic claims have been overstated, and controlled trial has shown it to be helpful only when depressive symptoms are definite.

Psychotherapy
Supportive type valuable. Insight-directed formal therapy difficult. Secondary gain may impede progress.
May need conjoint approach with spouse or 'key other'.

Behaviour therapy
Rituals. A significant proportion helped by response prevention. Admit to hospital, 24 hour monitoring, strong dissuasion, provision of alternative behaviour. Based on principle that repetition is a pathogenic factor in encouraging and consolidating rituals. Modelling involves the therapist touching feared objects, then encouraging patient to do so. Similar to flooding. Useful to carry out this approach in patient's home after discharge from inpatient care: involve family in modelling. Based on extinction process.

Obsessional thoughts. More difficult to treat, not amenable to behaviour therapy. Thought stopping involves encouraging to switch train of thought.

Leucotomy
Sometimes used as last resort when illness is severe and in danger of becoming chronic (2–3 years duration), good previous personality, no aggressive traits, physically well, absence of significant interpersonal or social causal factors. The 1983 Mental Health Act requires consent as well as a second medical and two non-medical opinions in all patients.

PROGNOSIS

Episodic course with remissions common. Basic amelioration rate: 66% fully well or much improved and leading normal life 5 years after onset. 79% illness episodes last less than 1 year (Pollitt).

Improvement may await changes in environmental perpetuating factors.

Rarely leads to development of psychotic illness: only slight increase in incidence of psychosis in relatives.

Predictors of poor outcome

Marked mood disorder (anxiety, depression, anger). Long duration of symptoms before treatment commenced. Reluctance to accept help.

FURTHER READING

Crowe, M. J. (1976) Behavioural treatment in psychiatry. In *Recent Advances in Clinical Psychiatry–2*. Ed. K. Granville-Grossman. Edinburgh: Churchill Livingstone.

Grimshaw, L. (1965) The outcome of obsessional disorder: follow up of 100 cases. *Brit. J. Psychiat.*, **111**, 1051–1056.

Rachman, S and Hodgson, R. J. (1980) *Obsessions and Compulsions*. New Jersey: Prentice Hall.

C. ANXIETY STATES

ICD9 DEFINITION

Various combinations of mental and physical manifestations of anxiety, not attributable to real danger and occurring either in attacks or as a persisting state. The anxiety is usually diffuse and may extend to panic. Other neurotic features such as obsessional or hysterical symptoms may be present but do not dominate the clinical picture.

EPIDEMIOLOGY

The most common neurotic syndrome. More common in women. Estimates of life time prevalence vary: up to 17 per 1000 in men and 38 per 1000 in women.

CLINICAL FEATURES

Important to differentiate normal day to day anxiety from neurotic symptoms which are disabling in some degree.

Useful to distinguish two components of symptoms.

1. Psychological

Sense of apprehension which may be focussed on specific threatening situations or only vaguely related to recognised fears, poor concentration (may lead to fear of memory impairment), irritability, hypochondriacal preoccupation, initial insomnia, sleep disturbed by fearful dreams. May be intermittent tearfulness and depression of mood but this is minor in degree relative to features of anxiety.

2. Physical

Motor restlessness, tension headaches, increased startle reaction, action tremor of hands.

Great variety of somatic symptoms referred to many systems:

Gastrointestinal: poor appetite, feelings of nausea, frequent bowel action, abdominal discomfort

Respiratory: overbreathing, feelings of difficulty in achieving adequate air intake

Cardiovascular: Palpitations, chest discomfort

Genitourinary: frequency and urgency of micturition, impotence and loss of libido.

Autonomic (sympathetic) overactivity: cold sweaty peripheries, fine tremor of hands, tachycardia, dry mouth.

DIFFERENTIAL DIAGNOSIS

Depressive illness. Look for specific depressive symptoms, early morning wakening.

Organic states such as dementia which may lead to agitation and secondary anxiety. Look for specific clinical features of organic brain syndrome.

Alcohol and drug dependence.

Physical illness. Anxiety may arise secondarily to an awareness of incipient physical disease. Thyrotoxicosis mimics anxiety states closely (look for marked weight loss with retention of good appetite, heat intolerance, warm peripheries with tachycardia and high sleeping pulse rate).

Rare conditions include phaeochromocytoma and spontaneous hypoglycaemia.

TREATMENT

Supportive therapy. Important to listen and provide personal support. Anxiety may reflect current life difficulties, and often subsides with them in time.

Medication. Beware of using high dosage and long courses of minor tranquillisers because of risk of dependence. Many patients remain on chronic low dose medication and this is undesirable. Do not prescribe benzodiazepines for longer than a few weeks.

Antidepressant drugs may be useful because of their anxiolytic effect particularly if prolonged medication is indicated.

Beta receptor antagonists. Limited value, but of some use when palpitations are troublesome.

Relaxation and Anxiety Management Training. Extremely useful. Allow patient to learn control of the self and lead to increased self confidence. Many patients prefer this approach to drugs.

D. PANIC ATTACKS

Recently suggested that these are a distinct form of anxiety disorder. Two kinds proposed:
1. Provoked by a stimulus that the patient recognises: probably an intense form of phobic anxiety. Avoidance response to exposure treatment.
2. Arises spontaneously. No avoidance response but may improve with imipramine. Debate whether this really is a separate entity (as suggested in DSMIII) or merely a very severe anxiety disorder.

Difference in symptom patterns difficult to interpret because some may develop secondary to the attack itself (especially somatic type fears). Some evidence that type 2 has a greater incidence of previous depressive disorder, and excess of panic disorder but not generalised anxiety disorder in first degree relatives.

CAUSAL THEORIES

Over-activity of the sympathetic nervous system. This may arise through heightened sensitivity of end organs (no significant experimental evidence) or increased activity in sympathetic nerves, possibly involving variable activity of the locus ceruleus in the fourth ventricle (as yet experimental evidence inconclusive).

Response to imipramine. Clinical trial evidence that imipramine may have specific positive effect in panic attacks. The aetiological implications of this are not yet clear.

Hyperventilation. This produces symptoms which resemble those of panic attacks. Likely that over-breathing may play a part in some attacks but there is no convincing evidence that this is a principal causal factor in the majority.

Abnormal cognition. Variable tendency of substances such as sodium lactate, caffeine to provoke panic attacks. Deliberate over-breathing may also act as precipitating factor. Psychological cognitive variables may account for individual differences in response to these precipitating factors. Treatment of panic attacks involving change of cognitions may be a useful approach.

E. PHOBIC ANXIETY

DEFINITION

A phobia is a special form of fear which is out of proportion to the demands of a situation, cannot be explained or reasoned away, is beyond voluntary control and leads to avoidance of the feared situation (Marks).

Usually many physical autonomic concomitants of anxiety.

CLINICAL TYPES

Related to external stimuli
Most common:
Agoraphobia 60%
Social phobia 8%
Animal phobia 3%
Miscellaneous specific phobias 14%

Related to internal stimuli
Illness phobia, hypochondriasis.
Obsessive phobias.

Agoraphobia
Commonest and most distressing. 66% are females. 6.3 per 1000 general population, onset 18–35 years of age. Fear of open spaces, often also for going out alone, into crowds, travelling, closed spaces.

Usually accompanied by diverse anxiety symptoms. Social anxiety common. Family often stable, closely knit.

History of childhood fears (night terrors), enuresis in 55%.

Sexual frigidity in 60% female patients (significantly more than control group). Less common in males: antedates or follows agoraphobic symptoms. Onset in some follows traumatic event with situational panic.

Avoidance of phobic situation may be marked, aimed at anxiety reduction.

Secondary involvement of family common.

Symptoms may serve secondary gain.

Associated non-phobic symptoms:
— general anxiety
— depersonalisation (37%)
— depression
— obsessional compulsive phenomena.

Specific animal phobias
Majority commence before puberty. Many remit as relearning occurs. Less likely to have multiple associated anxiety symptoms. Contrast agoraphobia.

Social phobias
May lead to gross restriction of social activities because of self conscious fears. Onset usually after puberty.

Illness phobias
Hypochondriasis (multiple fears). Nosophobia (fear of specific illness). May be symptomatic of other condition:
— lasting personality trait, e.g. obsessional.
— depressive or schizophrenic illness.
— response to anxiety or stress.
Previous health history or illness in relative may be relevant.

Obsessive phobias
Fear of contaminating or harming others or the self.
Repeatedly intrude into consciousness despite resistance.
No fear of the object, only the consequences therefrom.
Usually with compulsive washing, avoidance rituals.
Risk of acting-out fears is small in absence of significant depression or aggressive personality disorder.
Desensitisation difficult because extremely specific to each feared situation and little generalisation.

TREATMENT
Initial full assessment of the total situation essential.

1. Systematic desensitisation
Most effective in focal circumscribed phobias. Gradual exposure to phobic stimuli along hierarchy of increasing intensity. Practice in fantasy (imaginal) together with situational. Results superior to other methods. Benefits may accrue even in chronic agoraphobia. Problems may occur: achieving deep relaxation, providing vivid imagery of phobia, irrelevant/fluctuating hierarchy, lack of motivation due to life situational problems.
   Facilitated by: muscular and mental relaxation, expectation, reassurance, practice and suggestion by therapist, practice of regime, discourage avoidance behaviour, positive involvement of relatives. Poor response in agoraphobia, severe obsessions, high overt (free floating) anxiety with marked physiological correlates of anxiety.

2. Modelling (vicarious learning)
Observing model (therapist, relative) engage in non-avoidance behaviour with the feared stimulus.

3. Flooding (implosion)
In vivo or imaginal. Encourage maximal supervised exposure to feared stimulus as rapidly as possible until anxiety reduction is

experienced. Prolonged exposure may provide lasting
improvement, e.g. 4–5 hours over 2–3 days.

4. Paradoxical intention (logotherapy)
Seek out and encourage to expose self to phobic stimulus.

5. Relaxation techniques and hypnotic suggestion

6. Psychotherapy
Especially when other personality difficulties, secondary gain
present. May need conjoint therapy with relative. Commitment and
attitude of therapist important.

7. Drug therapy
Minor tranquillisers and antidepressants when relevant symptoms
severe. Avoid prolonged courses. Use in anticipation of situational
exposure.

NATURAL HISTORY, PROGNOSIS

Fluctuant course, tendency to relapse with panic attacks. If acute
situational precipitant, tends to clear gradually unless reinforced by
repeated trauma or when prolonged avoidance of feared situation
has occurred. When persistent for more than 1 year spontaneous
recovery unlikely. If secondary to depressive illness improvement
occurs as this remits. Agoraphobia tends to improve slowly without
treatment. Animal phobias do not. After desensitisation:
agoraphobia 45% much improved in 1 year. Other phobias 55%
much improved in 1 year. (Marks and Gelder.)

F. THE HYPERVENTILATION SYNDROME

The most common psychophysiological reaction due to anxiety
encountered by physicians (Pincus). Focusses anxiety on organs by
causing symptoms in them. Common in young females (29% of
those aged 15–30 years referred for neurological opinion).

SYMPTOMS

Faintness, visual disturbance, poor concentration.
Nausea, vertigo.
Fullness in head, chest, epigastrium.
Headache.
Breathlessness, palpitation, hot flushes, cold sweats.
Paraesthesiae, vomiting.

CAUSE

Calibre of cerebral blood vessels closely related to pCO_2 in blood.
Four minutes overbreathing can reduce cerebral blood flow by 40%.
Secondary alkalosis, tetany, fits.
May accentuate cerebral dysrhythmia in epileptics.
Exaggerated by orthostatic hypotension, valsalva manoeuvre.

DIAGNOSTIC TEST

Symptoms reproduced by 3 minutes overbreathing.

FURTHER READING

Boulougouris, J. C. & Marks I. M. (1969) Implosion (flooding). A new treatment for phobias. *Brit. Med. J.*, **2**, 721–723.

Gelder, M. G. (1986) Panic attacks. New approaches to an old problem. *Brit. J. Psychiat.*, **149**, 346–352.

Lipsedge, M. S. (1973) Systematic desensitisation. *Brit. J. Hosp. Med.*, (May) 657–664.

Marks, I. M. (1969) *Fears and Phobias*. London: Heinemann Medical.

Pincus, J. H. (1978) Hyperventilation syndrome. *Brit. J. Hosp. Med.*, (April) **19**, 312–313.

Watson, J. P., Gaind, R. & Marks, I. M. (1971) Prolonged exposure: a rapid treatment of phobia. *Brit. Med. J.*, **1**, 13–15.

Personality disorders

These are enduring aspects of psychological make up. Hazardous to make this diagnosis in adolescence or even in young adults because potential for major change is still present.

Adequate evaluation of premorbid personality facilitates assessment of a clinical problem by providing a baseline from which the following may be established:

Rate of development of illness
The extent of change from the normal self
Time relationship to environmental factors
Understand personal meaning of stress events.
Establishing realistic treatment goals.

PERSONALITY TYPES

ICD9 lists the following categories of personality disorders.

PARANOID

Either sensitive and blaming others or somewhat aggressive preoccupation with personal rights. In both there is an excessive tendency to self reference. There may be 'overvalued ideas' but no psychotic features such as delusions or hallucinations. Touchy and suspicious, does not make friends easily. May be jealous, stubborn, argumentative, litigious, prickly with inflated self evaluation, with a tendency to take offence and feel humiliation easily. May develop sensitive ideas of reference under stress, and these can be mistaken for persecutory delusions.

AFFECTIVE (CYCLOTHYMIC)

Persistent anomalies of mood-depressive, euphoric, or alternating between these.

SCHIZOID

Extreme reserve, shyness, aloofness, may be eccentric behaviour.

EXPLOSIVE

Instability of mood, liable to sudden irritability, anger, impulsive aggressive. At other times normal and not antisocial.

ANANKASTIC (OBSESSIVE COMPULSIVE)

Extremely cautious, conscientious, rigid, perfectionist, vaccilating and doubting, prone to anxiety depressive disorder. Inflexible, poor adaptability to change, excessively sensitive to criticism, often chronically resentful. Vulnerable to development of florid obsessive compulsive neurosis.

HYSTERICAL

Shallow, labile affective features, over-dependence on others. Erratic relationships, may be histrionic and may develop hysterical symptoms under stress.

ASTHENIC

Passive dependent, lack of resilience and mental vigour.

ANTISOCIAL (PSYCHOPATHIC)

Persistent antisocial behaviour with lack of sympathetic feeling or remorse. May be abnormally aggressive. Includes Psychopathic Disorder, defined under the 1983 Mental Health Act as a persistent disorder of disability of mind (whether or not including significant impairment of intelligence) which results in abnormally aggressive or seriously irresponsible conduct on the part of the person concerned.

The 1959 Mental Health Act included the phrase 'requires or is susceptible to treatment' but this caused problems: patient could be detained in hospital on grounds that treatment is required even though not susceptible to it. This wording was removed in the later Act, as was the age limit beyond which such patients could not be detained. Instead was added a treatability criterion, so that hospital detention only possible if treatment is likely to alleviate or prevent deterioration in the patient's condition.

Four key clinical features of psychopathic disorder
Failure to make loving relationships
Impulsive behaviour
Lack of guilt, callous, unfeeling
Failure to learn from adverse experiences.

Causes
47 XYY genotype in high proportion of psychopathic offenders: but probably only a few XYY individuals become persistently antisocial.

Immature slow wave pattern in EEG in up to 48% but interpretation requires caution (Hill).
May be no cultural background of criminality, but developmental environmental influences probably outweigh genetic ones.

Historical background
Phillipe Pinel (1801) Manie sans delire.
William Cowles Prichard (1835) described syndrome of 'moral insanity' characterised by 'morbid perversion of the natural feelings, affections, inclinations, temper, habits, moral disposition and natural impulses without psychotic features'.
Maudsley (1885) argued that offenders suffering from moral insanity were not fully responsible for their actions.
Henderson (1939) introduced the term 'psychopathic state' with three categories, aggressive, inadequate and creative.

Recent review concerning criteria for hospital treatment of antisocial personality (psychopathic disorder)
Working Group of DHSS and Home Office (Health Notice (86)28).
The current provisions for hospital detention are:
   Direct disposal to hospital by a Court (Section 37)
   Transfer from prison to hospital (Section 47)
   Remand to hospital by a Court for assessment
   An interim order before the Court decides on final disposal
   (Section 38).
If no special restrictions are imposed, then transfer or discharge may be decided by the Responsible Medical Officer, Hospital Managers, Mental Health Review Tribunal, or in certain circumstances by the nearest relative.
If Court imposes restrictions (Section 41) then discharge needs Home Office approval or on direction of a Tribunal.
   If restriction is from the Home Secretary, only he can decide on transfer or discharge, although Tribunal can advise.
   Problems identified by the Working Group:
   — Uncertainty regarding the concept of Psychopathic Disorder
      (its heterogeneity), treatability, and relationship with
      offending.
   — Difficulty in assessing amelioration and in predicting future
      behaviour.
   — Discharge of patients by Tribunals who judge them to be no
      longer suffering from Psychopathic Disorder to such a degree
      that hospital detention is appropriate, yet they still present a
      risk to the public (although such instances have been few in
      number).
   Options for change of Section 37 considered by the Working
Group:
   — Replace it by a procedure in which the Court passes a sentence
      but with immediate admission to hospital. As a result it would

not be possible for a Tribunal to recommend discharge, and subsequent remission to prison could take place should it be thought appropriate.
— Delete any reference to Psychopathic Disorder. In this case a Court would not have the option of hospital admission when this diagnosis applies.
— Hospital order only possible in Psychopathic Disorder in the absence of special restrictions.
Counterarguments against such changes:
— The problem is numerically a small one.
— The health disposal option for Psychopathic Disorder should not be reduced or made more difficult to arrange.
— Continuity of care would be broken by a return to prison.
— Improvement in hospital would be discouraged if it merely means eventual return to prison.

The Working Group's proposals have not received sufficient support and at present no specific proposals for change are being pursued.

BORDERLINE PERSONALITY DISORDER

This is included in the Diagnostic and Statistical Manual of the American Psychiatric Association (DSMIII).

Refers to persons who show instability in a variety of areas, including interpersonal behaviour, mood and self image. No single feature is invariably present.

At least five of the following are required:
— Impulsivity or unpredictability in at least two areas that are potentially self damaging, e.g. spending, sex, gambling, substance abuse, shoplifting, overeating, physically self damaging acts.
— A pattern of unstable and intense interpersonal relationships.
— Inappropriate intense anger, often poorly controlled.
— Identity disturbance: uncertainty about gender identity, goals, values.
— Affective instability: marked mood shifts (depression, irritability, anxiety, for hours or days).
— Intolerance of being alone.
— Physical self damage (suicidal gestures, physical fights).
— Chronic feeling of emptiness and boredom.

This category is not applicable to persons under the age of 18 years when Identity Disorder applies.

Under extreme stress transient psychotic symptoms may occur.

Evaluation of this concept. It is poorly defined and undoubtedly heterogeneous. It has not achieved wide acceptance outside the USA. Whilst randomised controlled trials have produced results which claim that in some borderline states symptoms may be alleviated by neuroleptic drugs, critics point out that clinical improvement is not marked and difficult to distinguish from placebo effect.

FURTHER READING

Davis, D. R. (1987) How useful a diagnosis is Borderline Personality Disorder? Leading Article. *Brit. Med. J.*, **249**, 264–265.
DHSS (1986) *Offenders Suffering from Psychopathic Disorder*. Health Notice (86)28.

Sexual disorders

A. SEXUAL DYSFUNCTION

ERECTILE IMPOTENCE

Types
1. *Total*. Neither psychic nor reflexive erections since puberty, or at the most only partial erections have occurred.
2. *Acute onset (primary)*. Erections may have occurred with fantasy or spontaneously but never successful sexual intercourse.
3. *Acute onset (secondary)*. Follows a period of normal potency and often related to traumatic event.
4. *Gradual onset (secondary)*. Following a period of normal potency, there occurs fall off in sexual interest and increasingly frequent erectile failure.

Causes
Type 1 is uncommon, possibly related to constitutional low sex drive. Type 2 and 3 often related to anxiety in sexual situation though may not have neurotic personality. Anxiety causes arousal above optimal for erection to occur when the optimal level is low, or there is negative correlation between arousal and erection. Type 4 has less obvious relation to anxiety which if present may be secondarily related to impotence. Tends to affect older men who have previous history of varying sexual interest. Sexual partner often the prime motivator in seeking treatment.

Psychological factors important in 90%, usually involving anxiety related to perceived threat in the sexual situation (e.g. due to poor sexual education, guilt and fear of discovery, punishment, loss of control, pregnancy). Depressive illness also important. Marked individual variation in cause of impotence related to level of anxiety, type of psychodynamic problem, vulnerability of potency mechanisms.

Secondary relationship difficulties frequently follow and the resulting hostility, estrangement and increased anxiety complicate the problem: attitude of sexual partner then becomes crucial and may be major perpetuating factor.

Organic factors important in 10%. Tend to give picture of persistent, progressive disability in contrast to psychogenic factors which tend to cause more variable disability, often related to specific situations.

Diabetes mellitus a common cause: 30–60% diabetic men have potency disorders. May occur when diabetes out of control; other possible factors include diabetic neuropathy, arteriosclerotic changes in penile vessels, hormonal and biochemical disorder and secondary psychogenesis.

Drugs causing impotence: adrenergic blockers, phenothiazines (especially thioridazine), imipramine (atropine like effects), MAOIs, minor tranquillisers. Alcohol excess a common precipitant.

Chronic debilitating disease, vascular obstruction of lower aorta, prostatectomy (rare and usually there is a preceding history of sexual dysfunction), temporal lobe disorders.

Endocrine disorders: adrenal and thyroid dysfunction.

Male climacteric (low plasma testosterone and high gonadotrophin) a dubious entity. Very uncommon cause of impotence, if at all. Castration, eunuchoidism, Klinefelter's syndrome, infantilism, ingestion of female hormones or antiandrogens. Relation between testosterone and impotence is complex. When impotence due to castration before puberty testosterone causes no improvement. Later onset cases occasionally respond to it but even when blood level of testosterone is initially low there may be little or no improvement.

PREMATURE EJACULATION

Persistent occurrence of ejaculation and orgasm against volition before the male wishes, before or immediately after penetration.

May date from adolescence or may be of later onset.

Sexual drive may be high or low.

May occur independently of erectile impotence or co-exist with it.

DELAYED OR ABSENT EJACULATION

Persistent absence of orgasm and ejaculation during coitus, in spite of normal desire and erection. Occasionally absence of ejaculation only ('dry run' orgasm) which may complicate use of hypotensive and major tranquilliser drugs or prostatectomy.

Delayed orgasm may be related to lack of drive due to sexual deviation or anxiety. May resemble gradual onset impotence with life long sexual hypo-excitability.

VAGINISMUS

Involuntary spasm of circular fibres of levator ani: in severe cases also the adductors of the thigh, erector spinae and glutei when sexual intercourse is attempted by male partner.

Causes. Usually a learnt maladaptive response. Fear of being hurt, possibly related to previous painful experience, long standing fear of intercourse, faulty sex education, sex equated with guilt. Vicious circle of failure, e.g. marital tension, accentuation of any potency problem husband may have.

Assessment. May show acute anxiety on digital vaginal examination.

FRIGIDITY

Impairment of woman's capacity for genital sensory pleasure or for any aspect of the emotional experience coincident with it. May be absence of orgasm, vulval anaesthesia.

Causes. Often but not necessarily reflects wider marital and/or personality problems. May be temporary after childbirth, related to fatigue, physical ill health, anxiety over day to day matters, depression, fear of pregnancy, dislike of contraception, coitus interruptus over prolonged period of time, lack of privacy. Secondary marital tension often perpetuates.

TREATMENT OF SEXUAL DYSFUNCTION

Important to provide adequate treatment for other related disorders.

Drugs
Variable effect of anxiolytics. Androgens of uncertain value in impotence: a small proportion of cases may respond to high dose depot preparation of testosterone, e.g. Sustanon 250 mg weekly.

Marital counselling
Use initially when wider conflict in marital relationship is paramount: include non-sexual issues.

Individual psychotherapy
If neurotic personality difficulties severe.

Behaviour therapy
Pioneered by Masters and Johnson who outline the principles of the New Sex Therapy as follows:

Physiological response such as erection, which itself cannot be consciously controlled directly, is not striven for per se: allowed to take care of itself.

Brief highly concentrated behavioural psychotherapy aimed directly at symptoms, e.g. daily sessions for 2 weeks.

The couple seen as a functioning unit through which treatment occurs. Joint responsibility for progress, neither being the primary patient.

Dual-Sex Therapy Team. Important to counter any tendency for one therapist to impose own personal values on the couple: permits fuller understanding of both male and female attitudes: controls any sexual element in transference.

Aim is to give pleasure rather than receive it. Clear goals at all stages.

Sequence in treatment. Basic education (anatomy/physiology), establish good communication, full discussion of sexual feelings, hostilities, resentments.

Sensate focus with ban on intercourse or genital contact. Mutual exploration to establish areas of pleasurable tactile stimulation. Primary aim is not own sexual gratification, couple freed from demands of responding sexually, and so 'performance fears' reduced. These lead to loss of spontaneity, a tendency to watch own performance (spectator role) and to self-validating fears when partner is seen to become less spontaneous.

Specific dysfunction dealt with after sensate focus established. In impotence allow female to play dominant role, avoid sudden switch from foreplay to intercourse. In premature ejaculation female masturbates partner to point just short of ejaculation, then squeezes glans between thumb and first two fingers (Seman's technique). Gradual assumption of sexual intercourse. Vaginismus may require initial relaxation and individual psychotherapy (may include use of dilators) before couple therapy can proceed.

PROGNOSIS IN SEXUAL DYSFUNCTION

Good outcome associated with previous adequate sexual function, acute onset impotence, short duration of disability, adequate heterosexual desire, free from other psychological problems, and absence of secondary estrangement.

B. SEXUAL DEVIATION

DEFINITIONS

Anomaly of sexual inclination and behaviour which is not part of a psychosis or other illness.

Homosexuality. Sexual attraction with or without physical relationship between members of the same sex.

Fetishism. Sexual excitation and gratification arises mainly or exclusively from inanimate articles somehow related to the human body usually of the opposite sex, often articles of clothing.

Paedophilia. Desire of adult to engage in sexual activity with children of either sex.

Transvestism. Sexual pleasure derived from dressing and sometimes masquerading in clothing of opposite sex.

Exhibitionism. Sexual gratification from exposure of the male genitals to females.

HOMOSEXUALITY IN THE MALE

37% males experience orgasm during homosexual behaviour at some time. (Kinsey USA 1948.)

Common, even regarded as normal in societies which do not prohibit it.

May be transient phase in adolescence.

Causes

Those that push individual away from heterosexuality.
Learnt inhibition (family attitudes, ignorance, fear of disease).
Incestuous feelings about mother or sisters.
Lack of confidence in own sexual potency, sexual identity.

Those that pull towards homosexuality
Need for security may dominate any sensual aspect of relationship especially when older male chosen.
Self esteem when not available through other relationship.
Fear of males causes erotic passive response (ethological parallels).
Material gain.

Congenital and prenatal
Increased concordance rates in twins (MZ pairs show greater concordance than DZ pairs).
Presence of androgen at critical pre and neonatal periods determine later masculine type of behaviour.

Environmental factors
Probably predominate in choice of gender identity. Abnormal relationship with parents: unsatisfactory or absent relationship with father. Close binding intimate relationship with mother who may behave erotically towards son, prefer him to husband, overprotect and discourage his normal heterosexual development.

Choice of regular homosexual identity may be related to secondary perpetuating factors which depend on how rewarding it continues to be. May retain both heterosexual and homosexual orientation. Latter may then be source of marked anxiety. Others completely identify with homosexual identity and adopt mannerisms and life style accordingly, ensuring its perpetuation.

Management

Establish clear aims and reasons for referral. Coercion not justified.

Treat concomitant problems (mood disorders, neurotic illness, social support). May prefer to continue with homosexual orientation: support accordingly.

Those who wish to become heterosexual; true motivation for change crucial and the amount of coercion from other must be evaluated.

Treatment focussed on four main areas: reduction of heterosexual anxiety, increase in heterosexual responsiveness, development of satisfactory heterosexual behaviour, reduction of deviant sexual interest.

40% show benefit from treatment.

Specialised techniques

Indication of good response include age less than 35 years, and the presence of some heterosexual interest at some stage in the past, absence of widespread personality difficulties and perpetuating attitudes. Treatment must be combined with regular review discussions.

Systematic desensitisation more effective than aversion in those who have obvious heterosexual anxiety. Aversion more effective when less general anxiety but some anxiety about homosexuality.

Encourage adoption of heterosexual social interaction and behaviour, in parallel with specific behaviour therapy. Other psychological difficulties may appear during treatment, e.g. depression, difficulty in relinquishing life style, realisation that sexual deviance has led to secondary gain (e.g. avoidance of social situation in social phobia).

Techniques of modification: aversion therapy involves association of noxious stimulus (emetics to produce nausea, electrical stimuli), with deviant stimuli or responses either mental or physiological (e.g. penile erection).

Modification of sexual fantasies by pairing them with imagined unpleasant mental images and by encouraging heterosexual masturbatory images.

Systematic desensitisation used when marked anxiety towards heterosexual situation present. Progression through hierarchy with relaxation. May involve Masters and Johnson principles.

Positive conditioning of sexual response using pleasant reward.

HOMOSEXUALITY IN THE FEMALE

2.2% of adult female population (England and Wales). Kinsey found 4% single women remained exclusively lesbian from 20–35 years of age. More often related to companionship than sexual gratification.

Lesbian relationships tend to be more stable than those between homosexual males. Increased vulnerability to episodes of depression, anxiety.

EXHIBITIONISM

The repeated exposing of the genitalia inappropriately to strangers.

Accounts for one third of all recidivist sexual offenders. Rarely associated with indecent assault or sexual violence. May signify increased risk of paedophilia or hebephilic tendencies, homosexual contact and voyeurism.

Not a clear cut syndrome: part of behaviour dominated by immature goals of genital display, inspection and manipulation. Tend to be timid and unassertive socially, though aggressive in own family. Suggest disorder in ability to handle and express aggressive impulses. Often complain of impotence, premature ejaculation.

Tend to be in two groups. The first: timid, inhibited, with much sexual guilt. May expose flaccid penis. The second: aggressive and sociopathic. Usually expose erect penis, often whilst masturbating. Sexual excitement increased by response of others.

TRANS-SEXUALISM

The wish to change sex, often with deep conviction that assignment to wrong sex has occurred.

Sustained feminine gender identification and wish to alter bodily appearance towards opposite sex.

Some heterosexual drive likely to be present if there has been a history of fetishistic arousal.

More common in men than in women. Passive homosexual male may seek sex reassignment to rationalise a relationship. 47XYY genotype may predispose to trans-sexualism.

Sex reassignment surgery. Used in a small minority of trans-sexualism (single, absence of antisocial behaviour, intelligent enough to adapt to change, over 21, must have irrevocable pattern of cross-sex behaviour).

TRANSVESTISM

The wish to wear clothing appropriate to the opposite sex, often associated with sexual gratification. Some resemblance to fetishism. Heterosexual drive predominates in 67%; homosexual in 33%.

Psychotherapy useful in supportive form but relatively ineffective in achieving radical change in sex orientation. Hormone therapy (oestrogens, antiandrogens in male). Aversion therapy possibly more effective in transvestism than in trans-sexualism.

INTERSEXUALITY

A state between normal male and normal female.

Causes

Chromosomal. (Turner's syndrome, triple X female, chromatin positive Klinefelter's syndrome 47XXY, double Y male 47XYY.)

Gonadal. (True hermaphroditism with both ovaries and testes, simple gonadal dysgenesis.)

Mullerian. (Disordered embryogenesis.)

Hormonal. (Adrenal hyperplasia at birth or later causing virilisation in female; early failure of foetal testes or failed response of target organ to androgens may cause feminisation in male. May also be due to tumours of testes, adrenal or pituitary glands, liver disease, administration of oestrogen.)

Diagnosis of sex at birth: apparent sex judged by genitalia (may be deceptive), nuclear sex (females have chromocentric or Barr body indicating 2 X chromosomes in buccal smear) chromosome analysis, urinary 17 ketosteroids.

SEXUAL OFFENDERS

Tend to be older than other offenders and to be of slightly lower intelligence. Recent increase in number of adolescent indecent exposers. Victim may play part in initiating episode and dictate its precise form by her subsequent reaction.

Exhibitionism

3000 convictions in England and Wales per annum. Rate doubled since World War 2 though that for adult men constant. Group therapy may help shy passive individuals. Systematic desensitisation of heterosexual anxiety also useful.

Rape

Sexual intercourse with a woman against her will, whether by force, fraud or intimidation. More than one third occur between acquaintances. Motives may range from misunderstanding in sexual situation to deeper hostility towards females. Alcohol abuse commonly related.

May require prolonged psychotherapy: group setting may be helpful. Hormone therapy when sex drive extreme. A woman who has been raped may suffer prolonged adverse sequelae such as anxiety, phobias, depression, sense of humiliation, disgust at sexual feelings.

Paedophilia

Children under 16 years not legally capable of giving sexual consent. (A man cannot give consent to homosexual act if under 21 years). Psychotherapy, especially group, behaviour therapy. In extreme cases hormone therapy.

Incest

Prior to 1908 this was not a criminal offence. Incestuous father may merely disregard normal sexual taboos, may be paedophiliac or may have other sexual psychopathology. Whole family may need to be treated.

Sexual violence

A proportion (22%) of long term prisoners have committed offence involving some kind of overt sexual activity. Tend to be more violent than remainder, though less recidivist.

Treatment of sexual offenders

Hormone therapy. Patient must be fully informed of risks and give signed consent. Needs to be well motivated, and only justified in disorders liable to cause serious social complications. Oestrogens may cause breast hypertrophy, testicular atrophy, osteoporosis (oral ethinyl oestradiol 0.01–0.05 mg/day causes least nausea). Depot preparation: oestradiol undecylenate 50–100 mg once every 3–4 weeks. Benperidol or butyrophenone and the antiandrogen cyproterone acetate also used.

Where possible treatment should be as a condition of probation. Criminal Justice Act 1972 allows this kind of treatment for up to 3 years, the patient remaining in the community.

FURTHER READING

SEXUAL DEVIATION

Armstrong, C. N. (1968) Intersexuality. *Brit. J. Hosp. Med.*, March, 667–673.
Bancroft, J. H. J. (1974) *Deviant Sexual Behaviour.* Oxford: Clarendon Press.
Gunn, J. (1976) Sexual offenders. *Brit. J. Hosp. Med.*, Jan., 57–65.
Randell, J. (1970) Transvestism and trans sexualism. *Brit. J. Hosp. Med.*, Feb., 211–213.
Rooth, G. (1973) Exhibitionism, sexual violence and paedophilia. *Brit. J. Psychiat.*, **122**, 705–710.

SEXUAL DYSFUNCTION

Bancroft, J. H. J. (1970) Disorders of sexual potency. In *Modern Trends in Psychosomatic Medicine 2*, ed. O. W. Hill. London: Butterworths.
Bancroft, J. H. J. Sexual dysfunction in men. *Medicine,* **30**, 1790–1792.
Cooper, A. J. (1970) Male sex dysfunction. *Brit. Med. J.*, **1**, 157–159.

Cooper, A. J. (1972) Endocrine impotence. *Brit. Med. J.*, **2**, 34–36.
Masters, W. H. & Johnson, V. E. (1970) *Human Sexual Inadequacy*. Boston: Little, Brown.
Masters, W. H. & Johnson, V. E. (1976) Principles of the new sex therapy. *Am. J. Psychiat.*, **133**, 548–554.
Spencer, E. Psychosexual problems in women. *Medicine*, **30**, 1793–1796.

Alcohol dependence

DEFINITIONS

Abnormal dependence a central concept. Initially this may be entirely psychological but it later progresses to physical dependence (i.e. true addiction) with biochemical changes at cellular level leading to withdrawal symptoms when alcohol intake reduced.

WHO (1952)

Alcoholics are those excessive drinkers whose dependence on alcohol has attained such a degree that it shows noticeable disturbance or an interference with their bodily and mental health, their personal relationships, and smooth economic functioning, or who show prodomal signs of such a development. They therefore need treatment.

Jellinek (1960)

... 'any use of alcoholic beverages that cause any damage to the individual or society or both'.

Chafetz (1974)

... 'any drinking behaviour that is associated with dysfunction in a person's life'.

Such definitions can be difficult to apply because the concept of disease entity is ill-defined, and they do not clearly delineate social from morbid use of alcohol. Addiction and harm are not synonymous: harm may occur without addiction, and true addiction may exist without obvious harm for long periods. Davies (1971) suggests definition of alcoholism as 'the intermittent or continual ingestion of alcohol leading to dependency (addiction) or harm.'

The alcohol dependence syndrome (WHO 1977)

This concept allows for a range of mild to severe dependence, relating to a complex interaction of both psychological and physiological factors. It is distinct from alcohol related disabilities. In the past there has been insufficient distinction between dependence and damage. An individual may be markedly dependent but not exhibit damage, and vice versa. Alcohol related harm should be assessed independently of dependence.

The syndrome has seven components:

1. Narrowing of drinking repertoire.
2. Salience of drink seeking behaviour. Other activities such as family responsibilities and work become neglected as drinking takes their place.
3. Increased tolerance towards alcohol.
4. Repeated withdrawal symptoms. Typically on waking, but subacute symptoms such as tremor and sweating may be experienced most of the time.
5. Relief drinking. Often in the mornings, to relieve withdrawal symptoms.
6. Subjective awareness of a compulsion to drink.
7. Reinstatement after abstinence.

EPIDEMIOLOGY

Prevalence
Early case detection difficult (failure of others to recognise, patient denial). About 400 000–700 000 alcoholics in UK (15–20 per GP). If include relatives, 1 in 25 closely affected by this illness (1 in 10 in Scotland and Northern Ireland).

Hospital admission statistics (England and Wales)
First admission: primary diagnosis alcoholism or alcoholic psychosis

1949	1952	1972	1985
434	2000	10 167	14 000

Partly related to increased services, though consistent with rise according to other indices such as the national drink bill, number of drunkenness convictions. Prevalence of alcohol cirrhosis increased by 163% since 1963. During the 1970s, deaths from cirrhosis and alcoholism both increased by 30%, and driving offences related to alcohol more than doubled, far exceeding increase in vehicle mileage. 1 in 3 drivers killed had excess blood alcohol. Breathalyser test introduced in 1967: immediate 11% fall in total number of road casualties and 15% fall in fatalities. This improvement has been ill-sustained in more recent years, probably related to drivers capitalising on the low chance of being caught.

Jellinek Formula $A = R(PD/K)$ where D = no. of deaths from cirrhosis, A = prevalence of severe alcoholism, P = proportion of cirrhotic deaths due to alcoholism, K = constant (0.695) derived from $C_1C_2/100$ (C_1 being % of alcoholics with cirrhosis, C_2 being % mortality among alcoholics with cirrhosis).

The formula estimates prevalence in England + Wales of 11/1000 general population though it has been criticised because K changes with time and varies from one community to another.

Prevalence surveys

	per 1000 gen. popn.			
	Male	*Female*	*Total*	
Medical & community agencies	6.2	1.4		Moss, Beresford, Davies
General practitioners			1.1	Parr
			2.0	Shepherd
			10.2	Wilkins

The more recent Wilkins survey included problem drinkers plus addicts, in central Manchester (high density population) and involved direct interviews with persons possessing 'at risk' characteristics who attended GPs.

Cohort studies	*Life expectancy of alcoholism*
Iceland (Helgason)	6–10% male; 0.4% female
Bornholm (Fremming)	3.4% male; 0.1% female

Interviews with representative sample of population (Manhatten USA) Prevalence 19/1000.

Of medical admissions to hospitals in UK: 18% (Moody 1976), in USA: 21–41% (Tamayo and Feldman 1978).

Sex
Male/Female ratio 4.3:1 (females may be detected less easily, and probably increasing incidence).

Age
Recent marked increase in young adults in Scotland.

Social class
In UK high in Class 1 in which cirrhosis also most common. In Italy, Sweden, some parts USA, most common in lower social classes. Lowest prevalence normally in middle class.

Occupation
High morbidity when there is ease of access to alcohol and its use is condoned. Morbidity increased × 9 in trade representatives of alcohol manufacturers and distributors. Special hazard in armed forces.

Ethnic group
High in Irish and North American Negro. Low in Jews.

Marital status
High in divorced, separated, widowers.

National alcohol intake
Correlates with higher prevalence in France than in Italy.
    50% increase in alcohol consumption in UK during the period
1960–1985. Close correlation between level of alcohol consumption
per head of population and convictions for public drunkenness;
drinking and driving; mortality from hepatic cirrhosis and hospital
admissions for alcohol dependence. Temporary fall of alcohol
consumption between 1979 and 1982 accompanied by reduction in
adverse effects, but upward trend has been resumed more recently
(RCPsych 1986).

Living conditions
Higher prevalence in urban than rural especially high living density.

CLINICAL FEATURES
Problem drinking
Arises out of social drinking. Great variation. Before onset of
physical dependence. Usually presents with social, interpersonal,
work, economic difficulties. Existence becomes increasingly centred
around alcohol, ensuring its availability. Increased alcohol intake,
especially symptomatic drinking at times of stress, and surreptitious
intake. May be episodes of acute drunkenness. Physical symptoms:
anorexia, nausea, diarrhoea, retching, especially in mornings.
Psychological symptoms: anxiety, depression, transient reversible
memory lapses for recent events (palimpsests), denial,
rationalisation, projection, regarding alcohol use. Resent
discussing it.

Addictive drinking
Jellinek distinguished 5 patterns of pathological drinking:
α — purely psychological dependence to relieve bodily or emotional
pain. No loss of control (i.e. able to curtail amount taken).
β — physiological complications e.g. cirrhosis but no dependence.
γ — loss of control, common in spirit drinkers. Can abstain.
θ — high tissue tolerance and withdrawal symptoms when attempt
to abstain. Otherwise may show no social disruption from drinking.
ϵ — spree drinking.
    Jellinek saw addiction as loss of control and/or inability to abstain.
    This classification criticised: deterioration through these
categories not inevitable. Loss of control a variable phenomenon
and may depend on availability of alcohol. It is not inevitable each
time alcohol is taken, and it is difficult to predict which drinking
episode will precipitate it.

COMPLICATIONS OF ADDICTION

Acute drunkenness

Highly likely when blood alcohol level more than 100 mg %. Some variation with level of tissue tolerance and rate of gut absorption depending on other stomach contents. More likely when some degree of brain damage present. Potentiated by other drugs such as barbiturates. If comatose, remember that this may be due to some other cause even though patient may smell of alcohol, and may be due to alcohol even when there is no smell of it.

Withdrawal symptoms

Onset 0–8 hours. Tremor, nausea, retching, sweating, vivid anxiety-provoking dreams. May proceed to delirium tremens (see below).

Alcohol tolerance

Initially increased, later impaired.

Psychological

Angry outbursts, disinhibited behaviour. Defence mechanisms.
    Anxiety, depression.
    Deliberate self harm, either non-fatal or suicide. The latter increased × 80 in male alcoholics (Kessel & Grossman). 16% life expectancy of suicide (Helgason).
    Cerebral atrophy: 70% may have radiological evidence especially frontal and parietal lobes. Detectable by psychometric tests in 58%.
    Delirium tremens. 48–72 hours after alcohol withdrawal, confusion, disorientation, gross ataxia, agitation, intense fear, visual/tactile hallucinations, paranoid ideation. Usually precipitated by relative or absolute alcohol withdrawal: concurrent infection common. Minor hallucinatory symptoms complicate withdrawal in 50% alcohol addicts, full blown DTs in 5%. Mortality from this 15% (infection, dehydration, injury, hyperthermia, circulatory collapse, status epilepticus).
    Alcoholic auditory hallucinosis: may be part of withdrawal syndrome, but may be independent of this, in setting of clear consciousness. Most last few days, a few become chronic. Uncertain relationship to incipient schizophrenia or dementia.
    Wernicke's encephalopathy: confusion, ataxia, nystagmus, internuclear ophthalmoplegia, disorder of conjugate gaze. Probably due to thiamine deficiency, acute degenerative changes in mammillary bodies, mid brain, brain stem. May lead to Korsakoff's psychosis with gross impairment of new learning and retention of very recent memory, occasionally complicated by confabulation.
    Morbid jealousy. May be related to impotence, rejection by partner.

Physical
Mortality 113% greater than expected. Increased incidence of respiratory disease, gastritis, peptic ulcer, acute pancreatitis, accidents, vascular disease (? related to hypertriglyceridaemia) neoplasms of larynx and upper digestive tracts, cardiomyopathy and heart failure. Nutritional deficiency, especially Vitamin B1. Early obesity, later weight loss.

Liver metabolism. Coenzyme NAD becomes reduced by alcohol dehydrogenase leading to rise in lactic and ketoacids. Acetaldehyde may be the cause of mitochondrial swelling after acute alcohol ingestion. Increased microsomal enzyme activity. Impaired gluconeogenesis (may cause hypoglycaemia after alcohol intake, usually when glycogen depleted). Reduced albumin and transferrin synthesis, increased lipoprotein synthesis, decreased fatty acid oxidation (fatty infiltration).

Alcoholic hepatitis. Usually after long history (10 years) alcohol abuse, precipitated by acute intoxication. Acute illness resembling viral hepatitis (pain, fever, jaundice), 10–30% die in hepatic failure, others may develop cirrhosis.

Cirrhosis. Hepatic fibrosis at early stage leading to portal hypertension. Occurs in 5–10% chronic alcoholics. 65% of all cases of cirrhosis are related to alcohol abuse. May develop encephalopathy (precipitated by haemorrhage, infection, sedatives, surgical procedures, protein intake). Oesophageal varices may be a major problem.

Neurological. Head injury, epilepsy, poly-neuropathy, (tender calves, impaired tendon reflexes, muscle wasting, sensory loss, unpleasant dysaesthesiae: probably caused by combined toxic effect of alcohol and nutritional deficiency), acute cerebellar degeneration, central pontine myelinoclisis (bulbar palsy, spastic quadriparesis, usually rapidly fatal). Marchiafava Bignami disease (intellectual impairment, fits, pyramidal signs, degeneration of corpus callosum), myopathy (acute or subacute with proximal muscle weakness), optic atrophy (methyl alcohol intake).

Foetal alcohol syndrome. Prenatal damage related to heavy alcohol intake by mother during pregnancy. Poor growth (67%), impaired intellectual development, facial changes, congenital defects 30–40%, neonatal mortality 17% (Hanson).

Family
Marital discord and failure. Children of alcoholic parents: increased risk of becoming alcoholic themselves later, marrying an alcoholic, developing other psychiatric problems. Alcoholics' wives: described as dominant, aggressive, masochistic, but no adequate control studies on this. Difficult to distinguish behaviour secondary to alcoholism in spouse from that which antedates it. Wives have increased incidence of alcoholism in own parents, and may have

married an alcoholic previously (? selective mating in some marriages). Occasionally connive with husband's drinking and in denying it. She may develop problems when husband becomes sober.

CAUSES

Social
Ethnic variation related to group attitudes as well as individual characteristics. Protection by identification of alcohol with religious ritual (Jews). Relevant factors: degree of group anxiety and acculturation, lack of social hierarchy or of alternative means of satisfaction.

Predisposing attitudes: alcohol use equated with masculinity, group solidarity and relaxation (as opposed to use with meals), symptomatic problem-solving use, ambivalent community attitude to alcohol.

National economic pressure: in France where many involved in alcohol trade the level of acceptable alcohol consumption high.

Personal
Genetic. High concordance in MZ twins (54.2% compared with 31% DZ), may be related to personality traits rather than specific genetic factors. No demonstrable antecedent metabolic defect demonstrated.

Psychological. Learnt habit: imitation, operant learning (social reward of anxiety reduction or prevention), classical conditioning. Imitation, identification may be relevant to increased vulnerability in children of alcoholic parents.

Personality: no single type. Often dependent, passive or anxiety prone.

TREATMENT

Early recognition: avoid stereotype of deterioration as synonymous with alcoholism.

'At risk' factors in patients attending GPs and probability of being alcoholic (Wilkins): 100% if previous drunkenness offence or ask for help with alcohol problem, 75% if smell of drink at consultation, 50% if peptic ulcer, gastritis, request sick note for symptoms which do not suggest physical illness, accident at home, live in hostel for homeless, 25% if work in catering or brewery trade, divorced or separated, single male over 40 years, history of marital dysharmony (Central Manchester).

Motivation: facilitate by education on effects of alcohol, confrontation, (e.g. ability to abstain), support, reassure and convey conviction that recovery possible, set realistic goals. Ultimate strategy may require removal of support which perpetuates pathological drinking.

The setting: out-patient management may be sufficient in two thirds of cases. In-patient treatment may be needed when withdrawal symptoms severe. Short stay (3 weeks) may be as effective as longer stay.

Detoxification centres in experimental stage in UK attempt to provide alternative to ineffective convictions for drunkenness. Referrals by police of persons drunk in public places.

Withdrawal symptoms: may need sedatives (chlordiazepoxide, chlormethiazole). Important to treat fluid, electrolyte and nutritional deficiencies. May need infusion of glucose and Vit. B. Watch for infection, prevent injury. Use anticonvulsants if fits occur, or previous history of these. Magnesium used by some centres to reduce CNS excitability.

Withdrawal regimes: diazepam in gradually reducing doses in the most popular. If it is to be carried out on an out patient basis, then drugs should be dispensed daily to avoid risk of overdose or misuse.

Dosage levels:

10 mg q.d.s. for 3 days
10 mg t.d.s. for 3 days
 5 mg t.d.s. for 2 days
 5 mg b.d. for 2 days.

Chlormethiazole. This is less satisfactory because of mounting evidence of its tendency to lead to dependence, and recent concern that it can cause fatal respiratory depression if taken with alcohol. A report from the Committee of Safety of Medicines (CSM 1987) estimates that there may be 50 deaths related to this complication in the UK each year. Chlormethiazole should only be used as a withdrawal regime on an in-patient basis, and not prescribed as maintenance therapy.

Dosage levels:

1.5 g t.d.s. for 2 days
1.0 g t.d.s. for 2 days
0.5 g t.d.s. for 1 day.

The addiction: individual, group, conjoint, family therapy. Commitment of therapist crucial. Previous claims of aversion therapy (apormorphine, emetine) difficult to evaluate (patient selection, high cost treatment). Antabuse useful in preventing impending relapse: reactions can be dangerous. Best to aim at total abstinence. Brief counselling may be as effective as prolonged therapy (Orford & Edwards).

Return to controlled social drinking: unlikely to succeed if physical addiction has been present.

Community services crucial: information centres and Councils on Alcoholism, hostels, social services, alcohol programmes in industry. Alcoholics Anonymous: mutual group supportive help emphasises cohesiveness, helping others, sharing of information and hope.

Prevention: Education on responsible use of alcohol, cost control of alcoholic drinks, responsible advertising, judicious use of restricted availability.

GOOD PROGNOSTIC FACTORS

Social stability, older, male, absence of psychopathic traits, cooperative attitude, amenable to change, first treatment, adequate intelligence.

FURTHER READING

Committee on Safety of Medicines (1987) *Current Problems No 20* (August 1987).
DHSS (1984) *Report of the Medical Working Group on Drug Dependence: Guidelines of Good Clinical Practice in the Treatment of Drug Misuse.* London: DHSS.
Royal College of Psychiatrists (1986) *Alcohol our Favourite Drug.* London: Tavistock.
World Health Organisation (1986) *Alcohol related disabilities.* Geneva: Offset Publications No. 32.

Drug addiction

DEFINITION

WHO (1969): a state, psychic and sometimes also physical, resulting from the interaction between a living organism and a drug, characterised by behavioural and other responses that always include a compulsion to take the drug on a continuous or periodic basis in order to experience its psychic effects and sometimes to avoid the discomfort of its absence. Tolerance may or may not be present. A person may be dependent on more than one drug.

LEGISLATION

Misuse of Drugs Regulations 1973
Notification of and Supply to Addicts

Drugs are dealt with in the four schedules. The regulations specify controls in the way more than 100 drugs in schedules two and three may be supplied to addicts. They require that the total quantity, or the number of dosage units should be specified both in words and figures. N.B. Drugs such as amphetamines and methaqualone, methyphenidate, phenmetrazine are subject to the same controls as opiates.

Require notification within 7 days by a doctor to the Chief Medical Officer, Home Office, of any person he has attended who is addicted to dextromoramide, diamorphine, dipipanone, cocaine, omnopon, hydrocodone, hydromorphone, levorphanol, methadone, morphine, opium, oxycodone, pethidine, phenazocine, piritramide.

Special licence required before a doctor can prescribe heroin, morphine, cocaine or any of their salts for treatment of addiction.

EPIDEMIOLOGY

Prior to the 1960s opiate dependence in the UK limited to relatively few who had been initiated through therapeutic contact with drug.

In 1960s explosive increase occurred in numbers who were addicted to heroin and cocaine, particularly in Metropolitan London. 500% increase by 1965. Younger persons, not initiated through therapeutic exposure. Social infection. Since then the total problem has continued to increase rapidly in size.

Number of addicts known to Home Office

Year	1970	1975	1983
TOTAL	1426	1954	10 235

First timers notified in 1983 exceeded those in 1982 by 50%.

Reliability of statistics appears poor because of failure to notify. Inadequate clinical assessment and reluctance to diagnose addiction common. Figures may under-represent the true situation by a factor of 5.

Most cases of opiate misuse aged 20–30 years, in which group the steepest increase in incidence has occurred. Male/female ratio 3 : 1. Trend towards increasing age of addicts in recent years.

Stereotype of the 'junkie' opiate dependent: social drop out, unemployed, preceding severe personality difficulties. Important to remember that this is the hard core of the problem: many probably use opiates only occasionally without social deterioration (chippers). Up to one third may eventually spontaneously stop drug misuse (Stimson).

Trend towards multiple drug misuse, for example a combination of barbiturates with opiates.

Use of cannabis widespread by young, middle class, above average educational attainment, perhaps leading normal lives without social misfit or psychological instability. Very different from the 'junkie' stereotype and without obvious immediate adverse effects (Plant).

Attenders at drug treatment centres often use opiates from illegal sources as well as from prescription. Thefts from retail chemists have become a major problem. Dipipanone (Diconal) abuse has increased progessively in recent years: proportion of addicts receiving it on prescription 2% in 1974, 6% in 1975 and 8% in 1976.

Increased mortality in young adults (× 28 expected) mainly related to intravenous misuse, usually involving opiates and barbiturates: may be due to drug overdose (accidental and related to loss of tissue tolerance, or deliberate and suicidal). Other indirect causes not involving lethal overdose also important (traffic or other accident, inhalation of vomit, burns, or in 5% septicaemia).

OPIATES (MORPHINE TYPE)

Now most commonly involves methadone, less often heroin. Cocaine may be used at the same time as a CNS stimulant though it does not produce tolerance effects. Intravenous administration of opiates common, leading to marked physical dependence and tolerance and high dosage, e.g. 300 mg of heroin per day.

In assessment important to search for injection marks and to carry out full physical examination. Frequently omitted.

Complications
Withdrawal symptoms. Craving, rhinorrhoea, agitation, anxiety, perspiration, tremor, diarrhoea, tachycardia. Influenza-like symptoms in mild cases.

Acute overdosage perhaps leading to coma (accidental or suicidal).

Infection. Phlebitis, septicaemia, acute bacterial endocarditis (beware recent onset cardiac murmurs), homologous serum jaundice, AIDS.

Cocaine abuse may cause paranoid state with hallucinations, visual or auditory, intense itching, tactile hallucinations of insects crawling on skin (formication).

Causes
Under-privileged background common with history of marked under-achievement. Resolution of frustration by developing group solidarity with others who are similar (Plant).

Management
Overdose. As for any coma. Nalorphine may precipitate severe withdrawal symptoms. Beware of ventricular fibrillation if cocaine is involved.

Withdrawal symptoms and detoxification
Severity of symptoms greatly influenced by psychological factors: fear of withdrawal may produce anxiety symptoms before physiological changes occur. Such anxiety is reduced when a basic contract is agreed and the patient is well supported during the withdrawal process.

Withdrawal as in-patient may be advisable in high dose opiate misusers, or those with other severe physical or psychiatric pathology.

The choice of drug is oral methadone mixture DTF (1 mg per ml). Note that this is 2½ times stronger than methadone linctus. There are no clinical grounds for using heroin or any other opiate as a withdrawal regime unless the patient shows an allergic reaction or other intolerable side effects of methadone.

The first step is to establish a baseline daily drug dosage for each patient: this is the minimum daily dosage that enables stabilisation without significant withdrawal symptoms. Most patients will need 20–60 mg of methadone per day.

Pharmaceutically pure heroin or morphine may be substituted by the same dose of methadone (but never exceeding 80 mg per day maximum), but street heroin is of variable purity and the assumed equivalent dose of methadone should be much smaller, usually in the order of 25% (see DHSS guidelines). Give methadone mixture DTF (1 mg per ml) in a dose of 5–10 mg orally 2–4 hourly until the patient is comfortable, alert and stabilised. The opiate need should be titrated against clinically manifest symptoms such as tachycardia, mydriasis, or perspiration rather than subjective psychological ones. After 72 hours the methadone daily baseline requirement can be calculated.

For in-patients a gradual withdrawal over a 6–10 day period may be appropriate for baseline doses of methadone of 10–25 mg daily. Baseline doses in excess of 25 mg should be lowered by 5 mg every 2 days until 25 mg is reached, then the 10 day regime is followed. A baseline dose in excess of 40 mg may require 3–4 weeks in hospital.

Out-patient/day patient. A more extended withdrawal regime may be appropriate.

Pink prescription forms EC10HP(AD) allow 14 days prescription for daily dispensing (2 days are supplied on Saturdays).

General practice. Categories of drug addiction best treated in general practice: intermittent drug misusers who are not physically dependent.
   — static 'therapeutic' addicts
   — opiate use less than one year duration, and not yet regularly injecting
   — need less than 40 mg of methadone per day.

Beware of possible gross exaggeration of daily dose requirements, and baseline dosage should never be more than 60 mg methadone per day.

The use of non-opiate symptomatic medication during detoxification for opiate drugs may be useful in some patients. Some may not need a specific methadone withdrawal regime. The following non-addictive drugs may be useful for symptomatic relief:
Promethazine (phenergan). Useful for mild physical withdrawal symptoms.
Propranolol (Inderal). Useful for high degree of somatic withdrawal anxiety.
Diphenoxylate. Especially valuable in controlling diarrhoea when this is a prominent withdrawal symptom.
Thioridazine. May be effective in low dosage in reducing anxiety during opiate withdrawal.
Benzodiazepines. Beware of their addictive potential. Preferably avoided, but if needed they should never be given for more than one month overall and always in small doses. Long acting forms, such as diazepam, may reduce risk of epileptic seizures in patients with a history of seizures in sedative withdrawal previously.

Treatment of the addiction
In the UK maintenance therapy permitted. Contrast USA where opiate addiction is regarded as criminal. Oral methadone preferable. Regular urine drug assay crucial. Current approach increasingly conservative and opiates used in treatment only as last resort for specific period of time. Need to monitor whether this approach will

lead to increase in illicit misuse of drugs. Intensive support over long periods essential in rehabilitation.

COCAINE

Euphoria, paranoid symptoms, stereotyped repetitive movements. Hallucinations. No physical tolerance and no withdrawal symptoms.

BARBITURATES

Increasing incidence, often involving intravenous route. Can cause necrotic skin ulcers. May be part of multiple drug abuse. Overdose leads to ataxia, dysarthria and dangerous coma. Withdrawal symptoms similar to alcohol when physical dependence is present: tremor, hallucinatory confusional state, akin to delirium tremens, fits. Drug withdrawal best carried out gradually in physically dependent individuals. Fits may occur within 2–3 days if dependent on short acting drug, but may be delayed for 10 days in the case of long acting barbiturates.

AMPHETAMINES

Cause stimulation, increased energy, euphoria, aggressive behaviour. Prolonged heavy abuse (more than 50 mg per day) may lead to paranoid hallucinatory schizophrenic-like psychosis: usually resolved when drug stopped, but occasionally becomes chronic. Withdrawal may be complicated by severe depression and suicidal risk. Methyl amphetamine often abused intravenously: vivid visual hallucinations common.

LSD

Not accompanied by dependence. Adverse effects include paranoid hallucinatory psychosis, acute anxiety, confusion, impaired judgement, disorientation. Recurrence may occur some weeks after intake stopped. Uncertain whether it can cause chronic psychosis. Chlorpromazine useful in severe reactions.

MARIHUANA (CANNABIS)

Widespread casual recreational use. No physical dependence. Causes euphoria, relaxation and sedation. Effects may occasionally be adverse, including depression, panic, distorted time perception, hallucinations, increased auditory acuity. Body image changes, disorientation, catatonic immobility, clouding of consciousness, change in sleep pattern. Chronic amotivational syndrome (apathy, reduced work performance). These probably more common in vulnerable personalities but they are unpredictable. May lead to errors of judgement, for example in driving. Users of marihuana are in general hostile to opiate abuse.

NICOTINE
Psychological and physiological dependence.

Types
Psychosocial (little nicotine intake and intermittent).
Indulgent (pleasurable oral reward).
Tranquillisation (usage often varies with emotional state).
Stimulation (to allay fatigue and maintain performance).
Addictive (to avoid withdrawal symptoms and maintain high levels of nicotine in the blood).

MISCELLANEOUS
Wide variety of drugs may become the subject of addictive misuse and constant surveillance required. Glue sniffing a recent example: may be complicated by liver damage.

FURTHER READING

DHSS (1984) *Guidelines of Good Clinical Practice in the Treatment of Drug Misuse.* Report of the Medical Working Group on Drug Dependence.
HMSO (1984) *Prevention.* Report of the Advisory Council on the Misuse of Drugs.

Mental handicap

DEFINITIONS

A condition of arrested mental development, to be distinguished
from dementia in which deterioration from a previously higher level
of intellectual function has occurred.

Handicap
A state of arrested or incomplete development of mind, which
includes handicap of intelligence and is of a nature or degree
which requires or is susceptible to medical treatment or other
special care or training.

Severe handicap
Renders the person incapable of living an independent life or of
guarding himself against serious exploitation, or will be so
incapable when of an age to do so.

These definitions emphasise general personality and social
functioning rather than I.Q. though handicap tends to correspond to
an I.Q. range of 50–75 and severe handicap an I.Q. below 50.

Mental handicap is relevant to the Mental Health Act 1983 only if it
leads to mental impairment.

PREVALENCE

Severe handicap
Prevalence 3.6/1000 general population. Usually declared at early
age, unable to acquire reading or writing.

Handicap
Prevalence more difficult to determine: criteria such as
employability unreliable (dependent on local economic conditions).
2–3% of population have I.Q. less than 70.

CAUSES

Severe handicap
Usually secondary to gross organic defects in central nervous
system due to following causes:

Genetic
   Autosomal dominant gene (e.g. tuberose sclerosis). 50% of
subsequent children are likely to stand at risk of inheriting the gene
and therefore being affected unless the gene has arisen *de novo* as a
new mutation. This is the case in 80–90% of patients with tuberous
sclerosis. When this occurs, subsequent children born to parents of
a person with this condition do not stand at increased risk.

   Autosomal recessive gene. Each parent is a clinically normal
carrier. Theoretical chance that 25% of children will be affected
(homozygous): 50% will be normal carriers (heterozygous): 25%
will be normal and completely free from the gene. Consanguineous
mating important predisposing factor.

   Sex-linked recessive gene. Males usually affected. Females
normal carriers. If mother is a carrier then approximately 50% of her
progeny are likely to inherit the gene: of these males will be
affected; the females are carriers.

   Chromosomal. Trisomy 21 (95% of Down's Syndrome and related
to failure of dysjunction during meiosis, associated with increasing
maternal age). 5% of Down's syndrome related to either
translocation involving chromosome 21 or mosaicism (non-
dysjunction after fertilisation).
   X-linked conditions may account for the excess of males among
persons institutionalised because of mental handicap.
   Fragile X syndrome (one fifth of boys with intelligence quotients
between 35 and 50 are retarded because of a gene on the X
chromosome, and one third of these are due to the fragile X
syndrome. Clinical features include large testes, high forehead, big
jaw, long 'bat' ears, large hands. The male fetuses of carriers can be
aborted and screening of relatives should be encouraged).
   XXY Klinefelter syndrome.

Intrauterine (prenatal)
The fetus is most vulnerable during the first 8 weeks of gestation
(embryonic period), when organogenesis occurs.
   Infective (rubella, syphilis, toxoplasmosis), metabolic (cretinism,
kernicterus due to Rhesus incompatibility), anoxic (ante-partum
haemorrhage), teratogenic agents (ionising radiation, anti-
neoplastic drugs, steroid hormones, anticonvulsants, coumarin

anticoagulants, organic solvent abuse, alcohol, cigarette smoking, and possibly lithium), maternal dietary deficiency (folic acid), maternal phenylketonuria, low birth weight (2500 g or less).

At birth, infancy, childhood
Traumatic (brain injury including nonaccidental type), infective (meningitis, encephalitis), anoxic, severe prematurity, post-vaccinal encephalitis (the pertussis vaccine has been the most implicated and this has now been omitted from the 'triple vaccine' as used previously), lead poisoning (especially children with pica).

Idiopathic
Probably the largest group. May be associated with gross anatomical CNS defects such as hydrocephalus, microcephaly.

Handicap
Not so commonly associated with organic CNS defects.
   In less severe forms it is a variation of the normal distribution of mental ability.
   All causes of severe handicap relevant.
   Social conditions causing lack of educational stimulus, may lead to apparent mild handicap which is susceptible to improvement.
   Handicap not associated with brain damage is far more common in lower social classes: this has been termed the subcultural type or educationally subnormal, probably directly due to social factors, and preventable.

CLINICAL FEATURES

The severely handicapped child does not acquire reading or writing.
May need hospitalisation to ensure adequate level of care and prevent self injury.
Ability to survive in community related to general personality development, especially affective warmth, as well as intellectual level.
Mild handicap may cause little functional impairment.
Secondary disability as reaction to handicap (e.g. emotional upset, aggressive behaviour) may be precipitated by educational misplacement.
Family may also show emotional upset caused by management difficulties.
Complications: failure in self care, antisocial behaviour (lack of moral sense, aggressive outbursts, especially when over-stressed or frustrated), exploitation by others, prostitution. In Down's Syndrome signs of premature ageing appear and Alzheimer-like changes in the brain with further intellectual changes appear in middle life.

INVESTIGATIONS

In infancy. Recognition and vigorous treatment of rhesus incompatibility and infections. Metabolic screening. Clinical assessment permits early recognition of mongolism.

School children. Regular assessment of intellectual capacity.

Differentiate from: childhood autism and psychosis, deafness, visual impairment and developmental aphasia.

The heterozygotes for some autosomal recessive conditions (e.g. phenylketonuria) in most cases can be detected by biochemical and specific enzyme assay techniques. This may involve assay of fetal cells obtained by amniocentesis. Parents who have already had a child with such a disorder should be alerted to the availability of prenatal diagnosis in subsequent pregnancies. Similar considerations apply to sex-linked recessive conditions such as Lesch-Nyhan and Hunter's syndromes in which heterozygotes (female carriers) can be identified by specific enzyme assay of cells. The sex of the fetus can be determined by chromosome investigation: termination of pregnancy may be offered when an affected male fetus is identified.

MANAGEMENT

Prevention
Genetic counselling, good obstetric and child care.
Early detection of parents liable to cause non-accidental injury.

Treatment
Should emphasise individual care and interpersonal contact.
Adequate opportunity and stimulus.
Small family-type units as opposed to custodial regimes.
Care in community preferable to institutional.
Day centre and training scheme integrated with local industry.
Adequate involvement of whole family, helping it to accept the handicap and to learn how to cope with it.
Educational psychologist has important advisory and treatment role.
Need close cooperation between family, social, educational and medical agencies.

FURTHER READING

Reid, A. H. (1982) *The Psychiatry of Mental Handicap*. Oxford: Blackwell Scientific Publications.
Russell, J. A. O. R. (1985) Mental handicap. In *Current Reviews in Psychiatry*, no. 1. London/Edinburgh: Churchill Livingstone.
Wiley, Y. V. (1984) *Mental Handicap*, 5th edn, eds Heaton-Ward, W. A. and Wiley, Y. V. Bristol: John Wright.

The Mental Health Act 1983: some important issues

DEFINITIONS IN THE 1983 ACT

Mental Disorder means mental illness, arrested or incomplete development or mind, psychopathic disorder and any other disorder or disability of mind.

Severe mental impairment means a state of arrested or incomplete development of mind which includes severe impairment of intelligence and social functioning and is associated with abnormally aggressive or seriously irresponsible conduct on the part of the person concerned.

Mental impairment means a state of arrested or incomplete development of mind (not amounting to severe impairment) which includes significant impairment of intelligence and social functioning and is associated with abnormally aggressive or seriously irresponsible conduct on the part of the person concerned.

Psychopathic disorder means a persistent disorder or disability of mind (whether or not including a significant impairment of intelligence) which results in abnormally aggressive or seriously irresponsible conduct on the part of the person concerned.

Note that:
 — The Act cannot be invoked merely for reasons of promiscuity or other immoral conduct, sexual deviancy or dependence on alcohol or drugs.
 — Mental handicap itself is no longer included, apart from those mentally handicapped persons who are included in a new category 'impairment' on grounds of abnormally aggressive or seriously irresponsible conduct.
 — Reference to treatability of impairment or psychopathic disorder is now removed from their basic definition, but is included in the criteria necessary for their compulsory admission to hospital.
 — Unlike the previous Act, there is now no age limit for detention of patients with psychopathic disorder.

COMPULSORY ADMISSION PROCEDURES

SECTION 2

Hospital admission for assessment (or for assessment followed by medical treatment).
Duration 28 days.
Application by nearest relative or approved social worker, either of whom must have seen the patient within 14 days of the application.
Medical recommendation: a) registered medical practitioner
                            b) recognised specialist in mental illness
These doctors should have examined the patient together or separately, in the latter case not more than 7 days should have elapsed between the two examinations.
    Patient has the right to appeal to a review tribunal within 14 days of admission to hospital.

SECTION 4

Hospital admission for assessment in emergency (when only one doctor is available and the degree of urgency does not permit delay for a second opinion).
Duration 72 hours from time of admission.
Application by nearest relative or approved social worker, either of whom must have seen the patient within the previous 24 hours.
Medical recommendation. Registered medical practitioner (if possible one who previously knew the patient, preferably the family doctor). The patient must be admitted within 24 hours of the examination (or of the application if made earlier).

SECTION 136

Removal by police officer to place of safety of persons who appear to be mentally disordered in a place to which the public have access, if in immediate need of care or control.

SECTION 3

Admission for treatment. The particular form of mental disorder must be specified, and it must be such that hospital admission is the only appropriate method of management.
    Grounds for application under Section 3 are
a) that the patient is suffering from mental disorder, severe mental impairment, psychopathic disorder or mental impairment, being a disorder of a nature or degree which makes it appropriate for him to receive medical treatment in hospital, and
b) in the case of psychopathic disorder or mental impairment, that such a treatment is likely to alleviate or prevent a deterioration of his condition, and

c) that it is necessary for the health and safety of the patient or for the protection of other persons that he should receive such treatment and that it cannot be provided unless he is detained under this section.

Duration. 6 months, renewable for six months, then one year at a time.

Application. Nearest relative or approved social worker.

Recommendation: registered medical practitioner with previous knowledge of patient as well as recognised specialist in mental illness.

SECTION 5(2)

Emergency detention of informal patient already receiving psychiatric care in hospital.

Duration 72 hours from the time when the report is furnished.

Application. The responsible medical officer (i.e. consultant psychiatrist in charge of the case.) A suitably qualified nominated deputy may act in place of the RMO. Patient may also be detained by a senior nurse (defined in the Act) for up to 6 hours until doctor arrives.

MENTALLY DISORDERED OFFENDERS

Remand to hospital for a report (Section 35)

If accused of imprisonable offence (including murder) or found guilty but not yet sentenced for such an offence (excluding murder). Court may remand a defendant at any time for medical and psychiatric reports to be obtained. Remand may be in hospital wing of prison, or bail with condition of residence in hospital. (In latter case there are no powers to detain if defendant decides to leave.)

The MHA1983 gives Courts a new power to remand an accused person to a specified hospital for a medical report to be prepared on the evidence of a doctor, provided the hospital agrees. The person is treated as an informal patient and the 'consent to treatment' provisions for detained patients do not apply.

Remand to hospital for treatment (Section 36)

If in custody awaiting trial before Crown Court or awaiting sentence for imprisonable offence other than murder. This is a new provision as alternative to remand in custody while awaiting trial, allowing treatment of serious mental illness. Requires suitable level of security in the receiving hospital. Has advantage of possible avoidance of the Court finding the accused person unfit to plead. The 'consent to treatment' provisions apply.

The court makes a hospital or guardianship order (Section 37)
Confined to offences punishable by imprisonment. Conditions are similar to those of Section 3 and the patient is subject to the 'consent to treatment' provisions for detained patients. Note that if the patient is suffering from mental impairment or psychopathic disorder it must be stipulated in the admission criteria that medical treatment is likely to alleviate or prevent a deterioration of the patient's condition (but not necessarily cure). Duration six months unless renewed for a further six months, then at annual intervals. The responsible Medical Officer assumes full responsibility for treatment and discharge except when a restriction order has been imposed by the Court: important recent debate and change in provision for these particular patients who under the previous Act could not themselves make representations directly to a Mental Health Review Tribunal (which is an independent body able to give an adequate judicial opinion). They could only request the Home Secretary to consider making such an application, and the MHRT could only act in an advisory capacity. The European Court of Human Rights recently concluded that the UK was in breach of the European Convention on Human Rights which provides that: 'Everyone who is deprived of his liberty by arrest or detention shall be entitled to take proceedings by which the lawfulness of his detention shall be decided speedily by a Court and his release ordered if the detention is not lawful'.

The European Court found that in England under the previous Act this did not apply, and stated that the only basis for continuing to detain a person on the grounds of mental illness was continuing mental disorder. The Law has therefore been changed with regard to patients on restriction orders and they may now apply directly to a Mental Health Review Tribunal for review of their detention.

Interim hospital orders (Section 38)
It can be difficult to make effective medical recommendations quickly and to predict whether an individual really will make good use of hospital treatment. Interim Orders allow further assessment, diagnosis and treatment in hospital for up to three months, renewable up to a maximum of six months, before the Court finally makes a decision. Applies to persons convicted before Crown Court of offences punishable by imprisonment (other than murder) and who suffer from mental illness, psychopathic disorder, mental impairment or severe mental impairment, and when there is reason to suppose that the mental disorder is such that it may be appropriate for a Hospital Order to be made.

Restriction orders

A Crown Court may decide to add further conditions to a Hospital Order with respect to restriction of eventual discharge of the patient from hospital, when it is considered necessary to protect the public from serious harm.

This is the Judge's decision, and he is the final arbiter on potential dangerousness, but he must receive evidence from one of the recommending doctors.

The effect is that the patient cannot be given leave of absence from hospital, be transferred or discharged by the Responsible Medical Officer, without the consent of the Secretary of State (Home Secretary). The Home Secretary can:

— Remove the restrictions if he thinks it appropriate
— Order the discharge of the patient, if necessary with certain conditions still in force, for example with regard to place of residence, probation supervision or attendance for psychiatric supervision.
— Recall a patient who has been conditionally discharged if deterioration in his condition occurs.

See also discussion re MHRT's.

CONSENT TO TREATMENT

Recently discussed in the Mental Health Act Commission Draft Code of Practice which makes the following points:
The rules of Common Law apply to all patients, whether informal or detained, except when Statute Law applies. There are three basic rules.

First Basic Rule. Any form of physical treatment applied without the patient's consent is a battery, unless the circumstances are such that his consent may be dispensed with.

Second Basic Rule. A patient's consent, to be effective, must be a real consent. It must be genuine, the patient should be able to judge the issue uninfluenced by coercion or by fraud or deception, and it must be based on sufficient information. In English Law this amounts to a description in 'broad terms' of the nature of the treatment proposed, its purpose, effects, likely side effects, awareness of possible alternatives and the likely prognosis without treatment. It should also allow for a possible change of mind.

Third Basic Rule. Anyone proposing to give any treatment to a patient is under a duty to use reasonable care and skill. This includes giving adequate information to the patient.

The 1983 Mental Health Act makes special provision for *certain treatments* which require consent:

1. Requires consent as well as mandatory concurring second opinion (Section 51) from a doctor appointed by the Mental Health Act Commission as well as two non-medical opinions. Only the doctor is expected to give an opinion on the validity of proposed treatment. This group of treatments concerns

hazardous and controversial methods such as leucotomy, stipulated under the Act and applies to all patients.
2. This applies to detained patients only. Requires consent or (if the patient is unwilling or unable to give consent) a second opinion. This must be given by another doctor who should consult a nurse and one other professional concerned with the patient's treatment. This group or treatments includes ECT and such medication and other treatments as may be stipulated in the Act. It does not apply to use of medicines (provided these are not in the 'limited' category) during the first three months following the first administration of medicines for the mental disorder, provided of course this falls within a period of time during which a patient is liable to be detained.

Urgent treatment
The above two conditions do not apply to any treatment
    : which is immediately necessary to save the patient's life
or : which (not being irreversible) is immediately necessary to prevent a serious deterioration of his condition
or : which (not being irreversible or hazardous) is immediately necessary and represents the minimum interference necessary to prevent the patient from behaving violently or being a danger to himself or to others.

The MHAC Draft Code expressed the view that consent is not required in the following circumstances (they have not been included in the more recent Draft Code of Practice issued by the DHSS because they are considered too complicated for application within a legislative framework).

Any patient, even in the Accident and Emergency Department, who is unconscious due to accident, overdose, or other physical disability. Any treatment is then lawful and proper without real consent if it is immediately necessary to save life, to preserve health from risk of serious deterioration unless there is a obvious risk of equal or greater deterioration as a result of the treatment being given.

The endangering patient, either concerning the life or health of others, or threat to harm himself.

The detained patient: medication during first three months of appropriate Order of the Act,
            : ECT, or medication beyond the three month period (but only if patient is incapable of giving consent or refuses to give it and a 'second opinion' doctor appointed by the MHAC has agreed).

MENTAL CAPACITY TO GIVE CONSENT

May be variable levels of ability: the lower the level the fuller the explanation required.

Incapacity usually associated with one or more of:
- mental handicap or organic brain syndromes, with global defect of reasoning and personality, sometimes with defect of memory.
- conditions in which judgement is impaired by delusions, irrational beliefs or the holding of mutually incompatible ideas at the same time, or by serious emotional disturbance or indecisiveness.

Detained status under the Mental Health Act does not by itself imply incompetence to give consent.

To be capable of giving or witholding real consent a person should be able to recognise:
- that he is clinically regarded as ill or handicapped and in need of treatment
- the problems consequent upon not having the proposed treatment.

The legal requirement for giving real consent is that the patient should be told in broad terms the nature and purpose of the treatment proposed (the responsible medical officer explaining it in simple terms), and so be able to understand its nature, its certain consequences and the serious risks attendant on it.

MENTAL HEALTH ACT COMMISSION

This is a multidisciplinary and independent body whose role is to exercise a general protective function in respect of detained patients. It visits hospitals regularly and appoints doctors to give second opinions. It also publishes an annual report and has some responsibility for informal patients.

MENTAL HEALTH REVIEW TRIBUNALS

These are independent bodies with lay, legal and medical members appointed by the Lord Chancellor. Allow review of patients' detention and provide right of appeal. There is now automatic referral to a MHRT. This did not occur under the previous Act, and many patients did not take the opportunity to have their detention reviewed. In such cases the 1983 Act now ensures periodic independent review of the need for continued detention by MHRTs.

Patients detained under Section 2 may appeal to a tribunal within the first 14 days. Those under Section 3 may appeal in the first six months and in the second six months, and then every year of detention.

There are new arrangements for the automatic review of a patient's case. Hospital managers are required to refer a non-offender patient to a tribunal for review after the first six months if the patient has not exercised the right to apply himself. A further automatic review must occur after 3 years if the patient has not requested one.

FURTHER READING

Buglass, R. (1984) *A Guide to the Mental Health Act 1983*. Edinburgh: Churchill Livingstone.

DHSS (1987) *Mental Health Act 1983. Draft Code of Practice*. Priority Care Division DHSS FA/2021b/46.

Mental Health Act Commission Draft Code of Practice (1985) Mental Health Division DHSS, Alexander Fleming House, Elephant and Castle, London SE1 6BY.

Mental Health Act 1983. London: HMSO.

Report of the Committee on Mentally Abnormal Offenders (The Butler Committee) 1975. London: HMSO.

Forensic psychiatry

CONDITIONS AFFECTING PERSONAL RESPONSIBILITY

1. AGE

Children under 10 years are not criminally responsible. From 10 to 14 children may be convicted if there is proof of mens rea and evidence that the child knew right from wrong.

2. MENTAL DISORDER

a) The Insanity Defence and The McNaughton Rules: Mens Rea (Guilty Mind) is absent because of the presence of mental illness.

The accused shall only be regarded as insane to the point of escaping responsibility for his criminal act if he was labouring under such a deficit of reason, from disease of the mind, as not to know the nature and quality of the act, or if he did know it, that what he was doing was wrong.

These are extremely narrow, and strictly would only apply to the severely subnormal or conditions such as delirium tremens. The rules reject the notion of irresistible or delusional impulses and are based on an intellectual test of responsibility. The 'Knowledge Test' can be very difficult to apply in practice: a psychotic illness may be severe yet not impair an individual's knowledge of his actions. Interpretation has been loose and variable. Used infrequently in recent years.

b) Diminished responsibility. Introduced in the 1957 Homicide Act. Provides that a conviction of murder will be reduced to one of manslaughter if at the time of the act the accused was suffering from such an abnormality of mind as to substantially impair his mental responsibility for the act. It thereby allows the sentence (for manslaughter) to be entirely at the discretion of the Court, and it may range from a hospital treatment order to a period of probation.

A wide variety of diagnostic categories has been included in successful pleas of diminished responsibility, including premenstrual tension.

c) Infanticide. Introduced in the Infanticide Act 1938. It applies to the period up to one year after the child's birth, and it has to be shown that the balance of the mother's mind was disturbed by reason of the effects of childbirth or lactation. Sentence is flexible.

3. AUTOMATISM

In legal terminology this means involuntary behaviour beyond the control of the person's mind. Non-insane automatism may lead to a full acquittal (e.g. sleep walking) whilst insane automatism (e.g. epilepsy) may result in committal to hospital without limit of time.

4. THE EFFECTS OF ALCOHOL OR DRUGS

Intoxication does not in itself constitute a defence. It may affect criminal responsibility:
— if it was such as to render it impossible to form intent
— if it caused a disease of the mind within the McNaughton Rules, e.g. delirium tremens.

INTENT

This is one component of guilty state of mind (mens rea) which needs to be proved in any successful prosecution. Intent means that the person perceives and intends that his act or omission will produce unlawful consequences.

FITNESS FOR TRIAL

If it is demonstrated that an accused person is insane and too mentally disturbed to be tried, he may be found 'unfit to plead' (or under disability).
Criteria of fitness to plead:
— understands the nature of the charge against him and the consequences of his plea of 'guilty' or 'not guilty'
— can follow court procedure, instruct his defence counsel and be able to object to the choice of individual jurors.

DANGEROUSNESS: CLINICAL POINTERS IN ASSESSMENT

HISTORY

One or more episodes of violence
Repeated impulsive behaviour
Difficulty in coping with stress
Unwillingness to delay gratification
Sadistic or paranoid traits
Chronic resentment

Mental illness: relapsing, poor cooperation
Head injury (disinhibiting effect)
Facility with weapons and access to them

OFFENCE

Bizarre violence
Unpredictable, lack of provocation
Lack of regret
Continuing denial
Intractable sexual deviancy of dangerous
    kind (paedophilia, aggressive fantasies or behaviour)

MENTAL STATE AND BEHAVIOUR

Morbid jealousy
Paranoid beliefs plus a wish to harm others
Violent fantasies if combined with other factors
Deceptiveness
Impaired insight
Lack of self control
Threat to repeat violence
Psychotic illness in which fear is significant
Poor attitude to treatment

CIRCUMSTANCES

Alcohol or drug abuse: continuing, reckless lack of control
Intractable social difficulties
Lack of support

SPECIAL CONSIDERATIONS IN ARSON

The underlying motivation can vary considerably and may include:
    Delusional states
    Revenge, anger, jealousy
    Cry for help
    Covering up crime
    Insurance fraud
    Political motive
    Gang activity for excitement (especially in juveniles)
    Desire to be seen as hero or feel powerful
Estimates of repetition in arson:
    30% repeat rate over 15–20 years
    High rate if element of fetishism, revenge, paranoid ideation or
    'irresistible impulse'
        Arsonists released from prison:
    — 20% long term offenders repeat in 5 years
    — 2% short term offenders repeat in 5 years

TESTAMENTARY CAPACITY (Ability to make a will)

Even though mentally ill, a person may be of sound disposing mind, the criteria for which are:
— understands what a Will is and what its consequences are
— knows the names of close relatives and can assess their claims to his property
— free from abnormality of mind that might distort feelings or judgement relevant to making the Will (delusional ideas may be disregarded if their content is irrelevant to the making of the Will)

Medical assessment should be based on interview with testator alone, although other key informants should also be seen to check accuracy of information.

PSYCHIATRIC COURT REPORTS (Trick and Tennent 1981)

The report should be concise, avoid jargon, and if technical terms are used they should be defined clearly.
The following sequence of headings is useful:
— Identification of the writer's present appointment, qualification, and whether approved under Section 12 of the Mental Health Act
— Place of interview and whether any third person was present
— Source of information
— Background details of the defendant
— If pleading guilty, defendant's account of the crime, attitude to it.
— Other behaviour including personality characteristics, abuse of alcohol or drugs
— Present mental state
— Mental state at the time of the crime. This is usually a retrospective assessment, and eye witness accounts are useful. Current psychiatric diagnosis may provide important clues, but not necessarily so. Even if judged to have been suffering from mental disorder, it is still necessary to assess the mens rea at the time of the crime.
— Fitness to plead
— Recommendations on treatment and disposal. Should be feasible (appropriate facilities available) and compatible with degree of dangerousness.

FURTHER READING

Briscoe, O. (1975) Assessment of intent: an approach to the preparation of court reports. *Brit. J. Psychiat.*, **127**, 461–465.
Grounds, A. (1985) The psychiatrist in court. *Brit. J. Hosp. Med.*, **(July)**, 55–58.

Gunn, J. (1977) Criminal behaviour and mental disorder. *Brit. J. Psychiat.*, **130**, 317–329.

Hamilton, J. R. & Freeman, H. (eds) (1982) *Dangerousness: psychiatric assessment and management*. Royal College of Psychiatrists. Gaskell Special Publication No. 2.

Scott P. D. (1977). Assessing dangerousness in criminals. *Brit. J. Psychiat.*, **131**, 127–142.

Trick, K. L. K. & Tennent, T. G. (1981) *Forensic Psychiatric Psychiatry: an Introductory Text*. London: Pitman.

Treatments

A. PSYCHOTHERAPY

INDIVIDUAL SUPPORTIVE

Indications
Useful in two groups of patient:
1. Those experiencing stressful circumstances.
2. Those with chronic psychological problems or mental illness.
   Aims:
   — to help them to achieve best adaptation possible
   — to reinforce existing personality structure and defence mechanisms.

Does not aim to achieve any radical change in personality or defence mechanisms.

Technique
Therapist adopts role of benevolent professional, fostering trust and positive expectations.

Permits patient to relinquish all or some of his self-reliance.

Dependent role sanctioned: patient need not feel shame or embarrassment.

Include in strategies:
— explanation
— encouragement, reassurance
— permission for catharsis
— environmental manipulation.

Basic rules:

Listen and say little. Avoid glib reassurance.

Do not interrogate. Encourage patient to be at ease.

Be empathic, accept patient non-judgementally.

Do not pronounce on general matters.

Avoid authoritative directions over what patient should do.

Avoid facile interpretations of behaviour and motives.

Keep own attitudes to oneself.

Do not over-identify with the patient (leads to excessive anxiety in therapist and impaired judgement).

Define aims clearly and the nature of help offered.

Set clear mutually agreed goals, frequency and duration of treatment.
Review progress regularly.
Respect confidentiality and avoid gossip.

Development of excessive dependency
The main complication. Liable to occur when therapist dominates and permits the patient too much passivity, fails to set mutually agreed goals from the start, or to review progress of therapy regularly.

FORMAL INDIVIDUAL PSYCHOTHERAPY: NON-DIRECTIVE (EVOCATIVE) PRINCIPLES

More intensive than supportive type, aims to achieve enduring personality change through a systematic scrutiny of the patient's past and present psychological life.
Promotes insight and encourages patient to discover answers himself.
Recollection and recounting of issues, feelings, situations.

Therapist interventions
Enquiry. Asking questions to elaborate patient's account.
Clarification. Pointing out and linking events so that patient is helped to understand repeated patterns in his feeling and thinking.
Explanation, interpretation. Offered as hypotheses for discussion. The precise content depends on theoretical model to be used. Occasionally used for the primary purpose of evoking emotional response (prokaleptic) rather than based on content validity.
Guidance of discussion. Ensure that emotionally painful but relevant topics are dealt with adequately rather than avoided.
Confrontation. Concerning inconsistencies, evasions and other defence mechanisms.

Therapist attitudes
Basic approach as for supportive therapy. In some variants, such as client-centred therapy, expression of therapist's own feelings is encouraged, together with 'genuineness, acceptance of patient with unconditional positive regard and accurate empathic understanding'.

FORMAL INDIVIDUAL PSYCHOTHERAPY: PSYCHOANALYTIC

A specialised form of non-directive (evocative) approach.

Freudian model

Therapist maintains a position of anonymity.

Techniques of free association: 5 daily sessions per week, each lasting 50 minutes.

Analyst interventions confined to elucidation of material, interpretation, confrontation, and reconstruction.

Analysand invests therapist with thoughts and feelings which originate from early experience. This is called the transference.

'Acting out' occurs when the transference affects behaviour outside the treatment situation.

Early interpretation requires a period of 'working through'.

Analysis of transference is central part of therapy.

Specific characteristics of a patient's transference reflect his psychopathology, and 'transference neurosis' develops when earlier neurotic components dominate his feelings towards the analyst.

Repressed material is thereby repeated in the present, though its relationship to earlier experience is not recollected: it is an illusory apperception.

Transference may include element of positive regard and emotional attachment, or hostility and rejection.

Patient-therapist interaction may also reflect other processes: e.g. habitual attitudes, personality traits and behavioural styles which are not specially a matter of transference.

Resistance leads to suppression of unacceptable mental contents, avoidance of topics in association, and distortion of unconscious impulses which appear in disguise: therapy includes analysis of resistances.

CONJOINT PSYCHOTHERAPY FOR MARITAL PROBLEMS

50% of marriages encounter early adjustment problems.

10% of married couples experience sufficient difficulty to contemplate or actually experience separation.

Most marital problems arise in first 2–3 years of marriage.

Divorce most frequent 6–7 years after marriage, and is particularly common when one or both partners married before 18 years of age.

Divorce Reform Act, 1969. Formulated grounds for divorce in terms of irretrievable marital breakdown.

The traditional marital offences (desertion, adultery, cruelty, incurable unsoundness of mind) are now mere components of more general evidence of breakdown, and their collusional manufacture is no longer necessary.

Fundamentals of conjoint therapy

Ideally:

— adequate motivation in both partners, with a genuine wish to improve the relationship and to continue with it, and a willingness to accept the need for personal change where necessary.
— neither partner is psychotic or so aggressive as to overwhelm the other in discussion.
— each must be able to represent own views but be prepared to see other partner's too and compromise where necessary.
— clear aims must be formulated and agreed by all concerned.

Therapist aims to:

— facilitate communication.
— avoid siding with one or other.
— avoid directing and advising.
— obey the rules of supportive psychotherapy.
— resolve conflict rather than encourage a quarrel.
— intervene to clarify, link aspects of behaviour or experience.
— confront over inconsistencies, or interpret.

Preliminary individual therapy indicated:

— when resistance to conjoint approach is severe.
— when one partner is initially too disturbed.
— when there is difficulty in sharing certain information.

Conjoint therapy essential to resolve relationship problems and avoids one partner being made into scapegoat. Can be useful in treatment of married individuals even when problems are not obviously related to marital relationship.

Points which may be revealed by conjoint approach:

— relative dominance of the partners.
— cooperation or scapegoating.
— style of decision making (one-sided or mutually agreed).
— use of defence mechanisms.
— respective behaviour in the partners (over-controlling, acting-out, or over-inhibited and self-contained, degree of self-reflection or conscience-directed attitude).
— relative view of marriage boundaries (e.g. extra-marital relations).

FAMILY PSYCHOTHERAPY

Based on the systems formed by individuals in families rather than focussed on individual psychopathology.

Indications

A family interview should be arranged when there is disorder of relationship, especially when the problem is not resolved by individual help.

Most useful when scapegoating and projective mechanisms marked.

Very disorganised families may need to be seen with other key individuals such as school staff.

Discussion of parental disharmony may act as reassurance for children, though it is inappropriate for them to be present when sexual problems of parents are dealt with.

Therapeutic processes
Variety of approaches. Therapist may direct, interreact or confront.
1. *Facilitation of communication*. Fundamental to all.
2. *Behavioural modification*. Learning theory principles.
3. *Psychoanalytic*. Deeper explorations needed when there is major resistance to change due to unconscious fantasies derived from childhood experiences. Transference already exists between marital partners, and therapist need not draw this on to himself. May be able to declare his own experiences (contrast individual therapy).
4. *General systems theory*. Based on principle that living systems are based on hierarchical sequence of supra and sub-systems which have boundaries between them. Within each there is a 'decider' mechanism. Resistance to change.

A family system needs a balance between open communication and sharing, versus separate autonomy of individuals within it.

Therapist may examine the way family resists change and tries to get him to collude in its psychopathology.

Outcome
Two studies suggest that short term crisis-orientated family therapy on out-patient basis is superior to conventional in-patient care (one quarter duration of disability, and time spent in hospital during subsequent 6 months may be halved). No significant difference in social and emotional functioning.

Spontaneous improvement occurs generally in family problems (66% in 2 years) but family therapy leads to more rapid resolution (86% in 1–3 weeks).

GROUP PSYCHOTHERAPY

Five to eight patients meet with one or two therapists for one and a half hour session each week.

May be closed group: no new members admitted.

open group: members who leave are replaced by new ones.

Based on process of learning by sharing experiences and caring for others.

Selection of patients
Able to express ideas and feelings verbally.

Can withstand exposure to group process and make use of interpretations.

Applicable in a wide range of diagnostic categories, especially neurotic and psychosomatic conditions, but selection must take into account the needs of the particular group.

May be preferable to individual therapy in emotionally deprived individuals because regressive dependency on therapist is less likely.

Members should be matched approximately in educational level and social class, but mixed in sex.

Patients who are unsuitable
Paranoid or psychopathic personality.

Psychotics.

Narcissistic or schizoid with little interest in others.

Extreme rivalry for attention.

Marked sensitivity to distress of others.

Basic group processes

First phase

Anxiety, defensiveness, ambivalence toward leader.

Establishment of group culture.

Trust established by exchange of self-revelation.

Individual styles become clear.

Second phase

Each member reacts individually to the processes of sharing, seeing the self in others, increased recognition of repressed feelings, and free exploration of associations.

Common themes are competitiveness, fear of exposure, sexual anxieties, dependency, autonomy.

Anti-therapeutic processes include scapegoating, development of sub-group alliances, group defensiveness, pressure to confirm and denial of differentiation.

Third phase

Before termination allow adequate working through of implications.

Some members may need further individual help.

Variants in technique

Bion

Traditional psychoanalytic: therapist confines remarks to interpretations in terms of group transference to therapists.

Whitaker and Leiberman
Confrontation of individuals as well as the group.

Foulkes
Allows interaction between members unrelated to transference to
therapist.

Encounter groups
Emphasis on the present, discourages exploration of past,
avoidance of concepts such as the unconscious or ego defences.
Therapist declares own feelings readily. As in T groups and Gestalt
therapy, the leader is active, directing, with inspirational charisma.
May involve physical contact between members of group.

Evaluation of group therapy
Complex and difficult: repertory grid technique useful.
   Truax: improvement in MMPI scores related to therapist empathy
and 'positive regard'.
   Vigorous therapist involvement with confrontation and challenge
may lead to ill effects in members who have low self-esteem and
high expectations of treatment.

B. CRISIS INTERVENTION

Caplan (1961) defines crisis as that which occurs when a person
faces an obstacle to important life goals that are, for a time,
insurmountable through the utilisation of customary methods of
problem solving. A period of disorganisation and upset ensues,
during which many abortive attempts at solution are made.
   Common problems tackled in crisis intervention: loss, change,
interpersonal, conflict.

Coping behaviours
   Problem solving
   Regression
   Denial
   Inertia
   Expression of affect.

Crisis
When coping behaviour fails, there are four possible phases of
crisis:
   Phase I   arousal and attempts at problem solving increase
   Phase II   due to excessive arousal, some impairment of function,
              disorganisation and distress
   Phase III emergency resources mobilised, novel methods of
              coping attempted
   Phase IV   failure to resolve crisis leads to deterioration and
              exhaustion.

Intervention

At an early stage it is necessary to decide whether to encourage autonomy and active coping (counselling), or whether decompensation indicates the need for urgent intervention and takeover of responsibility (intensive care).

Intensive care

Individual treated as sick and dependent.
   Transfer of responsibility to others
   Taking over immediate tasks, for example children's care
   Removal from stressful environment
   Lowering arousal and distress
   Reinforcing appropriate communication
   Showing concern, warmth, encouraging hope.
The aim is to reverse decompensation and restore normal coping as quickly as possible.

Crisis counselling

Individual is treated as someone who is asking for help and is able to retain responsibility for decisions.

   Nature of contract should be made explicit: objectives, duration and frequency of sessions, need for patients to accept responsibility for the outcome. Therapeutic techniques include:
   — Facilitating the expression of affect. Ventilation and full expression of feelings which are part of an understandable reaction to the crisis are usually beneficial. Their suppression may have damaging affects, for example suppressed anger leads to shocking or negative behaviour.
   — Facilitating communication of meaning. There may be longstanding difficulties in communication between relatives, rendering a family vulnerable at times of stress, or the crisis itself may impair communication.
   — Facilitating understanding.
   — Showing concern, empathy and bolstering self-esteem.
   — Facilitating problem-solving behaviour (define, identify and rehearse alternatives, provide expert advice, prescribe psychotropic drugs).

FURTHER READING

Bancroft, J. H. J. (1979) In: *An Introduction to the Psychotherapies*. Ed Bloch, S. Oxford: Oxford University Press.
Hobbs, M. (1984) Crisis intervention in theory and practice: a selective review. *Brit. J. Med. Psychol.*, **57**, 23–34.

C. THE THERAPEUTIC COMMUNITY

Social therapy (Milieu Therapy) is the use of the milieu as a mode of treatment.

HISTORY

Tom Main: Northfield Military Hospital, later at the Cassell Hospital.
Maxwell Jones: Belmont Hospital, later at the Henderson Hospital.
Units later at Claybury, Fulbourne, Littlemore, Dingleton and
Bethlem Hospitals.
Derivative approaches: Berne's Transactional Analysis, Perl's
Gestalt Therapy.

CHARACTERISTIC FEATURES

Permissive, egalitarian, democratic, communalistic.
Total resource, both staff and patient, pooled in furtherance of
therapy.
Patients are active agents of therapy and not passive recipients.
Small community, usually but not necessarily residential.
Reality confrontation, social analysis, face to face interchange.
Abolition of marks of differentiation such as titles, uniform.
Frequent total community meeting: regular daily and in crisis
situation.
Constant adequate communication throughout the whole
community.
Consensus decision making.

FURTHER READING

Clark, D. H. (1977) The therapeutic community, *Brit. J. Psychiat.*, **131**,
   553–564.

D. BEHAVIOUR THERAPY

INDICATIONS

Adults
   First choice in:
      — phobic disorders, social anxiety, obsessive-compulsive
         rituals.
   Useful in:
      — sexual dysfunction e.g. impotence, frigidity
      — sexual deviation e.g. exhibitionism
      — obsessive thoughts
      — habit disorders e.g. stammering, hair pulling, gambling
      — appetite disorders e.g. obesity, anorexia nervosa
      — social rehabilitation in chronic schizophrenia or organic
         defects.
   Not of value:
      — in acute schizophrenia, severe depression or hypomania
      — whenever clear goals cannot be worked out.

Children
First choice in:
   — nocturnal enuresis, phobias.
Useful in:
   — educational rehabilitation of subnormal children or those
   with learning problems, conduct disorders.

TYPES

1. Reduce anxiety-linked behaviour (phobias, compulsive rituals)
   by exposure treatment such as desensitisation or flooding with
   self regulation, modelling.
2. Reduce appetitive behaviour (e.g. exhibitionism, obesity) by self
   regulation, satiation, aversion.
3. Develop new behaviour (e.g. learn social skills) by training,
   education programmes, modelling, shaping, self regulation,
   prompting, pacing, feeding, contracting, contingent reward.

PRINCIPLES

Clear delineation of treatment goals.
   Patient cooperation essential.
   Family involvement when psychopathology involves relatives.
   Treatment taken to relevant settings, e.g. home, restaurants,
crowds.
   Inter-session home therapy by patient. Use of diary to rate anxiety,
behaviour practice in anxiety-provoking situations.
   May need to use more than one therapeutic strategy.

EXPOSURE TECHNIQUE

Can produce significant improvement in phobias or compulsions.
   Useful in social deficit and sexual dysfunction.
   Desensitisation in fantasy more rapid than with dynamic
psychotherapy, though long term outcome similar.
   Exposure *in vivo* for obsessive compulsive behaviour more
effective than relaxation therapy and benefit still marked at 2 years
(Marks 1976).

Techniques
Desensitisation. In fantasy only or *in vivo* by real life exposure to
phobic situation. *In vivo* probably more effective. Graded hierarchy
may not be essential.
Implosion. Exposure to maximal phobic situation until anxiety falls
and feel better, either in fantasy or in real life situation.
Modelling. Demonstration of anxiety-provoking behaviour by
therapist or relative.

Cognitive rehearsal and self regulation. Preparatory and concomitant reassurance, and techniques of self control of anxiety. *Response prevention.* In compulsive rituals.

Theoretical basis
Based on principle that given enough contact with the provoking situation, the phobic or obsessive person ceases to respond with avoidance, distress or rituals. Patients rarely become sensitised to a situation through exposure. Paradox that exposure to trauma sometimes produces phobias and for others is curative.

Some advocate anxiety reduction as essential in therapy (Wolpe), others maintain it is irrelevant (Marks). Implosion implies that maximal anxiety is required during exposure for improvement to occur.

Deliberate provocation of anxiety (more than inherent in exposure) is not more effective.

Long therapeutic sessions (2 hours) better than several shorter ones probably because it allows time for development of self regulatory strategies.

A small minority of phobic panics do not respond to exposure: some helped by antidepressants or abreaction (when fear irrelevant to phobic situation or anger present).

AVERSION TECHNIQUES

Used less often. Elimination of maladaptive response is of value only if replaced by more adaptive one.

The aversive stimulus is presented at the same time as the stimulus that elicits the undesired behaviour and leads to a conditioned anxiety response. Little empirical evidence for this.

Punishment training requires presentation of aversion stimulus contingent upon actual performance of undesired response.

'Covert sensitisation'. Training in imagining of traumatic consequences of problem behaviour as well as imagining the behaviour itself.

TOKEN ECONOMIES

Increase in contingency reinforced behaviour in psychiatric in-patients.

Problem of implementation:
rapid turn-over of ward staff
non-contingent reinforcement
maintaining effect after leaving token economy
enlisting patient's motivation.

CRITICAL EVALUATION OF BEHAVIOUR THERAPY

(American Psychiatric Association, Shapiro)
1. Based on experimental psychology. Caution in extending this to clinical situation.
2. Objective description and quantification of changes. May be unduly restricted to target symptoms.
3. Applicable to both psychological and organic illness. Need extreme caution in this approach to organic disease.
4. May help when psychotherapy has failed. Beware of placebo effect in evaluation.
5. Outcome evaluation used routinely. Rigorous criteria necessary here.
6. Experimental/control designs often used. True control can be difficult to define and obtain.
7. Claimed to be effective in many disorders: caution that claims do not outstrip the evidence. Behaviour therapy is a complex intervention and should not be over simplified.

E. DRUG THERAPY: SOME BASIC FACTS

(Specific dose regimens are not discussed, and can be found in relevant sections of the BNF).

PHARMACOLOGY

Amines important in central nervous system transmission.
The anatomy of the 'amine system':
   Distribution of aminergic fibres demonstrated by fluorescent microscopy.

5HT

Ho—[indole ring]—$CH_2CH_2NH_2$ Concentrated in midbrain raphe nuclei

DA

Ho—Ho—[benzene ring]—$CH_2CH_2NH_2$ Concentrated in substantia nigra, striatum, pituitary axis, arcuate nucleus of hypothalamus, limbic system

NA

Ho—Ho—[benzene ring]—$CH(OH)CH_2NH_2$ Clustered in brain stem near fourth ventricle

Differentiation of neurones containing noradrenaline (NA), dopamine (DA) and serotonin (5-hydroxytryptamine 5HT)

Amines are inactivated either by enzymatic action or by re-uptake into nerve terminals.

PSYCHOTROPIC DRUGS

Those which act upon psychic functions, behaviour or experience.

Antipsychotics (neuroleptics, atarectics, major tranquillisers)

Phenothiazines
Side chain — Dimethyl amino propyl (e.g. chlorpromazine)
— piperazine (e.g. trifluoperazine)

Thioxanthenes (e.g. flupenthixol)

Butyrophenones (e.g. haloperidol)

Diphenylbutyl piperidines (e.g. pimozide, fluspirilene)
May exert effects by inhibiting dopaminergic transmission through receptor blockade (note extrapyramidal side effects, experimental block of behavioural effects of stimulating nigrostrial pathway which contains dopamine, and reduction of evoked potentials in reticular formation from peripheral stimulation).

Two other drugs, oxypertine and sulpiride (N. F. 4.2.1.) may be useful where TD is present and antipsychotic therapy must continue. The current antipsychotic drug is tailed off, whilst commencing oxypertine orally 80 mg/day (to a maximum of 240 mg/day).

Unwanted side effects. Extra-pyramidal (EPS): Acute dystonia: includes facial grimacing, torticollis, opisthotonus, tongue protrusion. Can be controlled by biperiden lactate 2–5 mg intramuscularly (in severe cases, slowly by intravenous route) or benztropine mesylate 1–2 mg intravenously. May need to change the antipsychotic drug to one with different profile of action.

Akathisia: uncontrollable, unpleasant physical restlessness, often affecting the legs. Thiozanthines particularly associated. Treat by reduction of dosage level. Short course of a benzodiazepine may be helpful.

Parkinsonian syndrome: poverty of movement, rigidity, coarse static tremor, expressionless face. Treat with anti-Parkinsonian drugs, but beware of using these routinely as prophylactic because they may predispose to tardive dyskinesia or cause an acute organic syndrome. They may also retard the absorption of oral medication, augment its anticholinergic side effects, or be abused for their euphoric effect.

Tardive dyskinesia (TD): Involuntary facial chewing and choreoathetoid movement. A serious complication because it may not appear until several years after starting treatment; it does not necessarily improve with cessation of psychotropic medication, and sometimes gets worse when the drug is stopped. Develops in 20–40% of schizophrenic patients who have been treated with long term anti-psychotic drugs. Predisposing factors include: discontinuous treatment (regular drug-free intervals), increasing age, female sex, organic brain damage, past physical treatments such as ECT or insulin coma, defect state or Type II schizophrenic syndrome, intellectual impairment. May be due to drug induced dopamine receptor supersensitivity following prolonged dopaminergic blockade. Preventive measures important. Avoid long-term medication unless really essential.

In 50% the dyskinesia will disappear with reduction of level of medication, or its discontinuation if the mental state permits. Use of dopamine receptor agonists such as haloperidol or pimozide or dopamine depleting agents such as tetrabenazine, or oxypertine may be of value. Anticholinergic agents do not help and may even exacerbate TD. Claims that TD is more likely after long term high dose medication and use of anticholinergic medication have recently been challenged (Waddington and Youssef 1986).

Anticholinergic: Dry mouth, hesitancy of micturition, urinary retention, constipation, paralytic ileus, blurred vision, precipitation of acute glaucoma.

Antiadrenergic: postural hypertension, especially in the elderly, failure of ejaculation.

Miscellaneous: Drowsiness, galactorrhoea, amenorrhoea, hypothermia (especially in the elderly), reduction of seizure threshold, extra-hepatic cholestatic jaundice (chlorpromazine), skin rash and photosensitivity (especially chlorpromazine), SLE syndrome, cardiac arrhythmias, weight gain, retinal degeneration (thioridizine), agranulocytosis. Beware of use in first trimester of pregnancy (potential teratogenecity). Uncertain whether these drugs cause depression of mood.

Contra-indications. May potentiate opioid drugs, sedatives, alcohol. Avoid driving or operating machinery until dose is stabilised. Thioridizine may reverse the ionotropic action of digitalis. Pregnancy not an absolute contra-indication, but the drugs cross the placental barrier and appear in breast milk. If it is essential to continue drug treatment during pregnancy, change to the lowest possible oral dose of chlorpromazine. Infants may develop EPS.

Anxiolytic sedatives (minor tranquillisers)
Reduce pathological anxiety, tension and agitation, but no therapeutic effect on disturbed cognitive or perceptual aspects of psychosis. Cause little autonomic or extra-pyramidal side effects.

Benzodiazepines may lead to tolerance, physical dependence and withdrawal symptoms. In some (e.g. diazepam) the long half life may mean that withdrawal symptoms can occur up to a week after drug stopped. Can cause drowsiness, ataxia and occasionally (paradoxically) aggression.

Antidepressants
Affective illness may be due to failure in aminergic transmission. Antihypertensive drugs reserpine and α-methyldopa (which deplete the central nervous system of catecholamine derivatives) also may cause severe depression. It is not clear whether NA or 5HT involved.

Tricyclics
May act by blocking re-uptake process across the neuronal membrane through competition for NA receptors.

Side effects: dry mouth, urinary retention, constipation, confusion particularly in the elderly (anticholinergic effects), postural hypotension, drowsiness, blood dyscrasias, jaundice(rare), ECG changes (reduced myocardial conductivity and contractility, prolonged QRS interval), sudden death in patients with prexisting heart disease, glaucoma, epileptic fits (lower the epileptic threshold). Note that barbiturates and some anticonvulsants (phenytoin, carbamazepine, primidone) are enzyme inducers and will accelerate the metabolism of tricyclics.

Monoamine oxidase inhibitors (MAOIs)
Lead to striking rise in levels of 5HT and DA in brains of experimental animals. Should not be used at same time as drugs that block re-uptake of NA (e.g. amphetamine) or tyramine-containing foods (see p. 72) which release NA from sympathetic nerve terminals and may cause hypertensive crisis when taken with MAOIs.

MAOIs may also potentiate hypoglycaemia (caution in diabetics) and potentiate effects of morphine-like analgesics and anaesthetics (due to inhibition of hepatic enzymatic breakdown).

MAOIs may be most effective in depressive states that are not classically endogenous in type, where mood reactivity is retained, and there is high level of somatic anxiety, hypochondriasis, irritability, agoraphobia, obsessive preoccupations, panic episodes, histrionic behaviour.

L tryptophan
May be useful in treatment of depression when used in conjunction with MAOIs (rationale: its metabolite 5-hydroxyindole acetic acid levels low in CSF of depressed patients. Tryptophan is a precursor of 5HT).

Withdrawal syndromes in stopping antidepressants:
Gastrointestinal symptoms (excessive peripheral cholinergic
activation with abdominal cramps, vomiting, diarrhoea)
Insomnia, vivid dreams
Extrapyramidal symptoms (restlessness, akathisia)
Rarely hypomania, delirium, schizophreniform psychosis.

Lithium carbonate
Used as prophylactic in mania. Also of value in treating acute mania.

Prior to use check: cardiovascular, renal, hepatic and thyroid
functions.

Side effects: tremor, ataxia, abdominal distension, constipation,
vomiting, diarrhoea (when these develop, stop drug and check
serum levels), mild non-toxic goitre, hypothyroidism (block of
thyrotropic hormone), and diabetes insipidus. Fatal delirium, coma
in overdose: slow excretion hinders treatment (more than 95%
excreted via kidneys, hence beware of renal impairment).
Nephrotoxicity also possible.

Carbamazepine
Chemically related to tricyclic antidepressants and chlorpromazine.
Recently used to treat affective disorders, both in acute mania and as
prophylactic in both mania and depression. Further evaluation is
needed, but on present evidence it is reasonable to use
carbamazepine in manic depressive illness which is resistant to
conventional treatments. Maintenance dosage 600–1000 mg/day
(note that skin rashes may occur, as well as drowsiness, vomiting,
dizziness, increased toxicity of lithium).

FURTHER READING

Lader, M. (1980) *Introduction to Psychopharmacology*. Upjohn Scope.
Pare, C. M. B. (1985) The present status of monoamine oxidase inhibitors.
Brit. J. Psychiat., **146**, 576–584.
Waddington, J. L. & Youssef, H. A. (1986) Late onset involuntary movements
in chronic schizophrenia. *Brit. J. Psychiat.*, **149**, 616–620.

F. ELECTROCONVULSIVE THERAPY (ECT)

HISTORY

Early observation by mental hospital physicians: patients tended to
lose their symptoms when they had a spontaneous convulsion.
Epilepsy and schizophrenia rarely concurrent in the same patient.
Von Meduna 1935: induced fits using i.m. camphor in oil.
Cerletto and Bini 1933: electroshock first used.

PROBLEMS OF EVALUATION

Comparison of evaluative studies difficult because of heterogeneous patient groups and variation in diagnostic practice, failure to differentiate acute from chronic illness. Fully 'blind' control studies are rare (i.e. control involves giving anaesthesia without ECT) and ethically questionable.

EFFECTIVENESS

Depressive illness

Royal College of Psychiatrists Memorandum (1972) concluded that there is substantial and incontrovertible evidence that ECT is effective in severe depressive illness.

The most comprehensive studies suggest it is at least as effective as antidepressant medication, and quicker in action.

'Endogenous' type symptoms respond most readily but indication for ECT should be on basis of severity of depression and need for rapid response.

Status of unilateral versus bilateral ECT uncertain.

Two major early trials (random allocation of patients but not double blind)

Greenblatt et al, 1964. Multicentre, 281 depressed patients, 8-week trial period. Overall marked improvement with ECT 76%; imipramine 49%; phenelzine 50%; isocarboxazid 28%; placebo 46%. (ECT significantly better than any other at 1% level significance.)

MRC 1965. 269 patients with depressive illness as primary diagnosis. At 4 weeks nil or only slight symptoms: ECT 71%; imipramine 52%; phenelzine 30%; placebo 39%. At 4 weeks only female patients responded better to ECT than to imipramine and at 6 months the responses in the ECT and imipramine group were identical.

Some smaller studies have shown only minimal or no difference in effectiveness of ECT and antidepressants.

Double blind trials

Freeman et al 1978: Edinburgh. Placebo controlled. Bifrontal sinusoidal ECT twice weekly, compared with two simulated treatments in first week followed by real treatment. At end of first week the group receiving real ECT showed significantly greater improvement (on observer rating and one of two self report ratings) than control group. Subsequently the simulated treatment group required greater number of ECT applications.

Lambourne & Gill 1978: Southampton. Placebo controlled. Comparison of real and simulated brief pulse unilateral ECT applied ×3 weekly for 2 weeks. Both groups improved, and the only significant advantage of real ECT was in relief of hypochondriacal symptoms (although even this was regarded as fortuitous).

West 1981: Sutton. Cross-over design. Real compared with simulated ECT, twice weekly, bifrontal sinusoidal. Striking improvement with real ECT after 1 week, but no change in control group. Trial allowed patients not showing improvement after six treatments to be transferred to other group, and subsequently it was found that this option had been chosen in ten of the eleven patients who had started on simulated ECT, but in none who had commenced with real ECT. The ten 'switched' patients improved as soon as they received real ECT.

Johnstone et al, 1980: Northwick Park. Placebo controlled. Real and simulated ECT compared, total of eight applications twice weekly, bifrontal sinusoidal. Both groups improved steadily during treatment. At end of 4 weeks only modest advantage of real ECT, restricted to patients with delusions. At 1 and 6 months no significant differences between the two groups.

Brandon et al (1984): Leicestershire. Placebo controlled. Showed greater improvement in those patients given a full course of bilateral ECT compared with a simulated ECT group.

Possible explanation for different findings in these studies
Unilateral ECT used in Southampton study may be relatively ineffective form of treatment, and it may also have been difficult to be sure that bilateral convulsion occurred. Variation in patient selection may also have been important. Only 22% of Northwick Park patients had received ECT previously (compared with 55–66% in other studies) and they comprised 64% of all psychiatric in-patients admitted for treatment of depression. This very high proportion may explain why so many of the simulated treatment group recovered so quickly in this study.

   Long term outcome data, comparable to Northwick Park data, required in all studies if comparison is to be useful.

The Nottingham ECT study (Gregory et al 1985)
This replicated the methodology used by Lambourne and Gill, and in the Northwick Park studies. The findings suggest that both bilateral and unilateral ECT are highly effective treatments for depression, and significantly superior to simulated ECT. There was also evidence that patients receiving bilateral ECT recovered more rapidly, and required significantly fewer treatments, than those receiving

unilateral ECT. These authors suggest that the clinical choice of bilateral or unilateral ECT must remain a delicate balance between the need for a quick response, and the undoubtedly greater memory impairment produced by bilateral ECT.

Mania and hypomania
No satisfactory controlled studies. Some retrospective studies suggest that ECT leads to quicker and more complete recovery. The important question is whether ECT is better than drugs.

Schizophrenia
Recent study of Taylor & Fleminger (1980). Acute schizophrenia not responding to drugs randomly allocated to real or simulated ECT 8–12 applications. Significantly greater initial improvement with real ECT, but no difference at 16 weeks. It remains possible that longer course might have more lasting effect.

Generally agreed that ECT is of little value in chronic schizophrenia.

Unilateral versus bilateral ECT
Royal College of Psychiatrists Memorandum concludes that it is uncertain whether unilateral or bilateral ECT is more effective in depression. (In 29 studies, unilateral less effective in 13, identical in 14, more effective in 2.)

D'Elia and Raotmo suggest that non-dominant unilateral ECT has the same antidepressant effect as bilateral but causes fewer side effects such as memory impairment.

Some suggest that bilateral ECT acts more quickly in severe depression and few applications needed, but others disagree.

MORTALITY OF ECT
Surveys estimate 3–9 deaths per 100 000 ECT applications. (Compare mortality dental OP anaesthesia 0.3 per 100 000.)

Before ECT introduced, mortality in severe depressives 15% in 10 year period.

Recent 3 year follow up of 519 depressed patients showed much lower mortality in those who had received ECT.

Cholinergic effects of muscle relaxants may lead to serious cardiac dysrhythmias, and routine use of atropine to block this is imperative in ECT.

MORBIDITY DUE TO ECT

Immediate:
- — headaches and temporary confusion.
- — memory loss for recent events, diminishes rapidly after the final application but may increase with the number used.

Long term:
- — no objectively demonstrated memory impairment.
- — patients who have received bilateral ECT, subjectively rate memory as impaired 6–9 months later more frequently than do those who received unilateral ECT.

May be minor permanent loss of memory limited to events shortly before the time of treatment: effect increases with number and frequency of treatments and more likely with bilateral rather than unilateral ECT. Not likely to occur if treatment frequency is two or less per week.

'Kindling' phenomenon: sporadic grand mal fits for first time in the weeks or months after ECT rare, and do not persist over more than one year.

ECT induces extensive EEG changes: bilateral paroxysmal delta waves subside rapidly after treatment completed, and EEG usually returns to normal within three months.

TECHNIQUE OF ADMINISTRATION

Preparation
Full physical examination imperative.
Any significant organic disease discussed with general physician, anaesthetist.
Particular caution with cardiovascular disease (especially valvular).
Contraindications: recent cardiac infarction, severe pulmonary disease.
Ensure: availability of all medical/nursing notes at time of treatment.
- — resuscitatory equipment.
- — nursing staff.
- — overnight fasting.

Treatment
Anaesthetic given by anaesthetist (atropine, thiopentone, scoline).
Beware of prolonged paralysis due to pseudocholinesterase deficiency.
Oxygenate well before ECT given, and afterwards until normal breathing is re-established.
Avoid sub-convulsions: cause headache and anxiety.
Use least possible amount of current (memory disorder proportional to the amount used).

Machine should have choice of wave form and automatic timing.
If no convulsion, repeat application up to maximum of 3.
Electrodes placed over fronto-temporal areas in bilateral treatment
(some claim that memory is less impaired if placed over frontal or
occipital areas).
In unilateral treatment electrodes placed on mastoid and temporal
regions of same side.
    After convulsion:
        — patient is oxygenated with airway *in situ*.
        — patient remains under anaesthetist's supervision until
          spontaneous respiration returns and regains consciousness.
        — close nursing supervision in ECT room (watch for respiratory
          difficulties, cardiac arrest) and later in recovery room when
          reassurance and explanation important.
        — allow rest for about 1 hour.
    Usual number of treatments 6. Given regularly, usually twice
weekly.
    Little justification for daily application: probably increases
memory disturbance.
    Monitor response regularly.
    Antidepressant drugs may prevent relapse after treatment
stopped and reduce number of applications needed.
    A report to the Royal College of Psychiatrists recommends: a
consultant should be responsible for each ECT clinic, teaching and
training junior staff in the theory and practice of ECT, should be
personally involved in the clinic and ensure adequate standards.
    Need to improve standard of ECT facilities. Each clinic should:
a) specify the type of stimulus to be used, placement of electrodes,
procedure to be followed if first stimulus fails to produce a fit, and
the way atropine is to be used.
b) keep a patient register (name, date of attendance, number of
ECTs in present and past courses, complications).
c) keep a separate card index on each patient with details of
treatment, anaesthetic, relaxant, electrode position, stimulus, effect.
d) ensure that full case notes are available, and that the anaesthetist
is aware of the obligatory physical examination, current drug
therapy and drug sensitivities.
e) ensure that both a written account of what ECT involves as well
as verbal explanation is given to the patient and, where appropriate,
to relatives.
f) use only up to date safe equipment: Ectron Constant Current
apparatus and Series 4 machines (After 1979).
g) titrate length of treatment (number of applications) against
clinical response.

MEDICO-LEGAL ASPECTS

Fully informed written consent: both doctor and patient should sign to the effect that explanation has been given. Applies to both informal and detained patients. Single consent adequate for each course of treatment but patient may withdraw consent at any time.

Two doctors should be present when ECT given, one experienced in anaesthesia.

If patient unwilling to have ECT or unable to understand what is proposed, consultant reconsiders alternatives.

If ECT essential and considered safe, then a Treatment Order (Section 3) is needed to proceed and except in an emergency a written second medical opinion is required stating that although consent cannot be obtained, ECT is necessary in order to alleviate or prevent deterioration. Two other professionals concerned with the patient must also be consulted (one a nurse).

FURTHER READING

Brandon, S. et al. (1984) Electroconvulsive therapy: results in depressive illness from the Leicestershire trial. *Brit. Med. J.*, **288**, 22–25.

D'Elia, G. & Raotmo, H. (1975) Is unilateral ECT less effective than bilateral ECT? *Brit. J. Psychiat.*, **126**, 83–89.

Freeman, C. P. L., Basson, J. V. & Creighton, A. (1978) Double blind controlled trial of ECT and simulated ECT in depressive illness. *Lancet*, **i**, 738–740.

Gregory, S., Shawcross, C. R. & Gill, D. (1985) The Nottingham ECT study. *Brit. J. Psychiat.*, **146**, 520–524.

Johnstone, E. C. et al. (1980) The Northwick Park ECT trial. *Lancet*, **ii**, 1317–1320.

Kendell, R. E. (1981) The present status of electroconvulsive therapy. *Brit. J. Psychiat.*, **139**, 265–284.

Lambourne, J. & Gill, D. (1978) A controlled comparison of simulated and real ECT. *Brit. J. Psychiat.*, **133**, 514–519.

Pippard, J. & Ellam, L. (1981) Electroconvulsive treatment in Great Britain: a report to the College. *Brit. J. Psychiat.*, **139**, 563–569.

Royal College of Psychiatrists (1977) Memorandum on the use of ECT. *Brit. J. Psychiat.*, **131**, 261–272.

West, E. D. (1981) ECT in depression: a double blind controlled trial. *Brit. Med. J.*, **282**, 355–357.

G. PSYCHOSURGERY

HISTORY

1936 Moniz. Division of frontal lobe white matter to quieten aggressive behaviour. Awarded Nobel Prize 1949.

1942 Freeman and Watts. Standard leucotomy extensively used until early 1950s. At least 10 000 performed in UK between 1942–1952. (66% chronic schizophrenia, 33% affective illness.

Usually chronic illness with severe behaviour disorders prior to neuroleptic drug era.)

Imprecise, blind operation, serious complications common (apathy, flat affect, euphoria, disinhibition, aggression, intellectual impairment, incontinence, epilepsy, metabolic disorders).

Early 1950s advent of neuroleptic drugs, and leucotomy virtually superceded.

Subsequently, limits of drug therapy clear. Renewed interest in leucotomy (restricted, involving stereotaxis which permits precision in size and site of lesion).

Lesions used include cold, heat, cutting or electrical stimulation.

NEUROANATOMY AND NEUROPHYSIOLOGY

Profound autonomic and emotional changes induced by artificial stimulation of limbic system and amygdala.
Frontal lobe monitors and modulates limbic mechanisms.
Fronto limbic connections (4 main pathways):
— dorsal convexity via cingulate gyrus to hippocampus
— dorsal convexity to hypothalamus, mesencephalon
— orbital surface to septum
— orbital surface to hypothalamus.
Psychosurgery aims at:
— fronto limbic connections and where these are concentrated, viz, in the lower medial quadrant and posterior orbital area of the frontal lobes and the cingulate gyrus
— limbic circuits
— the limbic core.

EFFECTIVENESS AND COMPLICATIONS

Lesions of anterior cingulate gyrus
Electrical stimulation under local anaesthesia and stereotactic techniques used to aid target location (Kelly).

Claimed to be particularly effective in obsessional neurosis, especially when anxiety and depression prominent. Less effective in depression alone.

Lesions of ventromedial frontal lobe
These include bifrontal subcaudate tractotomy using Yttrium 90 isotope implant (Knight), orbital undercutting or bimedial operations (Schurr).

Particularly useful in severe depression, agitation and tension. Recovered or much improved: 60% depressives, 40−60% anxiety states, 50% obsessionals.

No affective blunting, reduced incidence of suicide attempts.

Lesions of amygdala or temporal lobes
Temporal lobectomy in:
— epileptics with aggressive outbursts (Turner).
— drug resistant epilepsy, when focal disease confined to non-dominant temporal lobe or the anterior 5–6 cm of the dominant lobe. Abolish fits in 50% when underlying lesion is mesial/temporal sclerosis, less effective in other disorders.

INDICATIONS FOR PSYCHOSURGERY

Advised by its exponents: in obsessionals, depression and anxiety states when other therapy has failed and illness relentless, disabling, becoming chronic.

When good previous personality and absence of psychopathy.

Free from organic brain and cerebrovascular disease.

Based on assumption that gross abnormality of limbic function may lead to intractible depressive, anxiety or obsessional neurosis.

Aims to restore neurophysiological balance without altering personality.

Not now used in schizophrenia unless above symptoms predominate.

Not acceptable as a way of controlling antisocial behaviour unless this is complication of relevant psychiatric disorder (e.g. temporal lobe epilepsy).

The Mental Health Act 1983 requires that in all cases of proposed leucotomy there should be concurring second medical and two non-medical written recommendations, as well as fully-informed consent.

When social/interpersonal factors are relevant to the illness, psychosurgery should not be undertaken until these have been fully treated and are clearly intractible. Insufficient attention to this point in recent literature. Psychosurgery should never be considered unless intensive and if necessary prolonged in-patient treatment has explored all other alternatives, including attempts to resolve intractible socio-economic and interpersonal difficulties.

REHABILITATION

Careful nursing supervision: monitor mood swings and suicide risk, retraining to avoid return to obsessional habits and to establish new routines.

FURTHER READING

Bridges, P. K. & Bartlett, J. R. (1977) Psychosurgery, yesterday and today. *Brit. J. Psychiat.*, **131**, 249–260.
Kelly, D. (1976) Neurosurgical treatment of psychiatric disorders. In *Recent Advances in Clinical Psychiatry–2*. Ed. Granville-Grossman, K. pp. 227–261. Edinburgh: Churchill Livingstone.

Special topics

A. SUICIDE

DEFINITION

WHO (1968): a suicidal act with fatal outcome.

Beck (1976): a wilful self inflicted life threatening act which has resulted in death.

STATISTICS

Assessment of intent difficult:
- — ambivalent motivation frequent.
- — often has to be inferred in absence of explicit evidence.

International comparison difficult: variation in categorisation, which may be carried out either by medical or legal personnel.

In some countries proof of intent (e.g. a note) is required before a death is classed as suicide. Otherwise open verdict recorded.

Official statistics may under-estimate incidence of suicide: in Dublin perusal of psychiatric records suggests true incidence 4 × official rate (McCarthy & Walsh).

If open verdicts are mainly concealed suicides, then official statistics are 22% too low.

High rank-consistency in suicide rates of various countries and of London Boroughs over prolonged period of time, irrespective of the individual coroner involved.

In the UK and USA suicide accounts for 1% of all deaths.

AGE, SEX

Incidence increases with age.

More common in males than females in all age groups.

In England and Wales: suicide rate in 1978 was 8.2 per 100 000 persons over 15 years of age.

Compare rate of 15.1 per 100 000 in 1962.

During period 1901–1970: marked fall in rates for older males, the male:female ratio falling from 3:1 to 3:2. The overall downward trend continued until 1975 when the rate for males was the lowest in this century. Subsequently, the suicide rate in England and Wales increased annually, from 7.5 per 100 000 in 1975 to 8.8 per 100 000 in 1980 (an increase of 17% overall, 21% in males, 12% in females). Since 1974, the sharpest rise has occurred in adults aged 25–44 years. Also a substantial increase in males aged 75–84 years. The fourth commonest cause of death in young adults. 1 in 800 000 age group 10–14 years. Extremely rare in children under 10 years old.

URBAN/RURAL

Urban rates greater than in rural areas but in recent years the difference has been less marked.

MARITAL STATUS

Incidence greater in divorcees, widows, widowers, than in single or never married.

SEASON

Highest incidence in April, May, June in northern hemisphere; during period spring to mid-summer in Australia.
   Seasonal variation more marked in females.

SOCIAL CLASS

Highest in Class V (unskilled).
   Moderate increase in Class I (professional) and IV (partly skilled).
   Lower than expected in Class II and III (lower professionals and executives, skilled manual and non-manual).

ETHNIC AND RELIGIOUS GROUP

Rates previously low in black Americans, but recent increase in young black suicide to level of whites.
   Relation to religious persuasion complex. Durkheim's finding of greater incidence in Protestants than Catholics not universally applicable today.

METHOD

In England and Wales since 1963: remarkable drop in number due to domestic gas, related to reduction of carbon monoxide content of town gas. About one third suicides due to this early 1960s, falling to near zero in 1972.
   Increase in drug poisoning (67% female, 37% male) particularly due to antidepressants, tranquillisers and salicylates.

Fall in barbiturate poisoning, though this was still the cause of 27% of all suicides in 1973 in England and Wales.

Violent method more common in males.

Use of firearm much more common in USA than in UK.

In England and Wales remarkable increase in suicide rate by motor vehicle exhaust during 1975–1980 (increase in males 75%, in females 64%). Also 47% increase in use of firearms by males. In 1985 only 8% suicides due to overdose of psychoactive drugs. Physical methods (hanging, gassing) in up to 51%.

CORRELATES OF SUICIDE

Age over 40 years. Male more often than female. (Age factor becoming less pronounced.)

Widowed, divorced, separated.

Immigrant.

Live alone, poor social contact and support.

Unemployed, retired.

Live in socially disorganised area.

Family history of affective disorder, suicide, alcoholism.

Previous history of affective disorder, alcoholism.

Previous suicide attempt.

Early in treatment for depression or soon after discharge from psychiatric hospital.

Addiction to alcohol, especially when significant complications present.

Incapacitating terminal illness in elderly.

Bereavement, separation, loss of job.

Personality: cyclothymic, sociopathic.

Mental illness:
- — severe depression
- — alcoholism, other addictions
- — early dementia
- — organic brain syndromes (epilepsy, head injury).

Symptoms:
- — depressed mood, persistent insomnia, loss of interests, hopelessness, self blame, agitation or retardation, social withdrawal, suicidal thoughts.

Attempted suicide:
- — precautions taken to prevent discovery, elaborate preparation, violent method or use of more lethal poison.

MANAGEMENT AND PREVENTION

Recognition of high risk groups

Suicide occurs in:

11–17% of severe (psychotic) depressions

7% of epileptics who also have organic brain syndromes

2% of schizophrenics
drug addicts at 50 × rate in general population
severe physical illness (a factor in 29% of suicides).
Note the danger of certain drugs which cause depression (reserpine, depot phenothiazines, barbiturates, contraceptives).

Difficulties encountered in the assessment and management of patients at risk of suicide
Deliberate denial of suicidal ideas.
Variability in degree of distress.
False improvement (removal from stress factors that remain unresolved).
Uncooperative and difficult behaviour.
Malignant alienation.
False assumption:
— that suicidal ideas which are openly admitted are usually manipulative threats which do not signify serious risk
— that direct discussion of suicidal ideas should be avoided for fear of increasing the risk.
Physical hazards in hospital wards or surroundings.
Poorly planned rehabilitation (misjudging the rate at which change can be expected or ignoring critical situational stressors).
Lack of clear plan concerning level of nursing observation.

Psychotherapy
Recognition and support for individuals in crisis especially the severely depressed.
    May need hospital admission or regular supportive help.

Physical treatment
Recent study showed that 82% of suicides were receiving prescribed psychotropic drugs at time of death (Barraclough et al, 1974).
    Irregularities in their use included:
— failure to use antidepressants specifically for depressive illness
— use of too low doses
— continued for many months
— excessive prescription of barbiturates and phenothiazines
— use of depot phenothiazines in non-schizophrenic illnesses
ECT needed in severe depression when immediate suicide risk severe.

Community services
In USA Suicide Prevention Centres developed.
In UK emphasis on voluntary agencies in collaboration with statutory services.
The Samaritans shown to attract high risk individuals.
Relative decline in suicide rate in towns where they operate (Bagley 1968). Interpretation difficult because of many other potentially

relevant social factors. Negative findings in more recent study (Jennings).

FURTHER READING

Barraclough, B. et al. (1974) A hundred cases of suicide: clinical aspects. *Brit. J. Psychiat.*, **125**, 355–373.
Jennings, C. (1978) Have the Samaritans led to a reduction in the suicide rate? *Psychol. Med.*, **8**, 413–422.
Lancet (1978) Leading article: Suicide and the Samaritans. *Lancet*, ii, 772.
McClure, G. M. G. (1984a) Trends in suicide rate for England and Wales 1975–1980. *Brit. J. Psychiat.*, **144**, 119–126.
McClure, G. M. G. (1984b) Recent trends in suicide amongst the young. *Brit. J. Psychiat.*, **144**, 134–138.
Morgan, H. G. & Nowers, M. P. (1986) MRCPsych Tutorial no. 4. *Brit. J. Hosp. Med.* Supplement, 13–17.
Roy, A. (ed) (1986) *Suicide*. Baltimore: Williams and Wilkins.
Sainsbury, P. (1973) Suicide: opinion and fact. *Proc. Roy. Soc. Med.*, **66**, 579–587.

B. NON-FATAL DELIBERATE SELF HARM (DSH)

(parasuicide, attempted suicide)

DEFINITION

A non-fatal act in which an individual deliberately causes self injury or ingestion of a substance in excess of any prescribed or generally recommended therapeutic dose (Kreitman).

A deliberate non-fatal act, whether physical, drug overdosage or poisoning, done in the knowledge that it was potentially harmful, and in the case of drug overdosage, that the amount taken was excessive (Morgan).

Recent definitions attempt to avoid interpretation of whether conscious intent of self destruction was present, because this is difficult to detect reliably and many episodes are not associated with conscious ideas of suicide.

INCIDENCE

Massive increase during the 1960s and early 1970s throughout the western world. At all ages, except the elderly, rates in females exceeded those in males by 1.5–2.5:1. Highest rates in late adolescence and young adults. Since the mid-1970s rates in males have fallen by 18%, and those in females by 25% approximately. In 1984, the overall rate in females was 400/100 000, in males 200/100 000. Self-poisoning the most common emergency medical admission in females, and second to ischaemic heart disease in males.

METHOD

Drug overdosage in 93% (psychotropic drugs 49%, barbiturates 14%, salicylates 17%).

In London nearly 50% of episodes seen in hospital accident departments involve more than one drug.

78% use prescribed drugs (67% their own, 11% other persons).

Hypnotic overdose more common in older patients, tranquillisers in 20–34 year age group, and analgesics in young adults (79% of those age 15–19 years who resort to DSH).

Recent alcohol intake within preceding 6 hours in 50% male and 25–45% female DSH patients.

Self laceration:
  — in 5–10% of those attending hospital.
  — a few are males who are severely depressed and inflict single deep coarse incision near vital point.
  — majority are females with delicate, superficial and multiple incisions, less commonly associated with overt depression.

Repetition of DSH in 25% males and 23% females in year after episode.

CORRELATES

Marked difference in incidence according to living conditions: high in central disorganised urban areas, where overcrowding, lack of amenities are marked and high proportion of population unskilled. Also high in local authorities council housing estates. Low in middle class areas (professional, managerial, skilled artisan).

Important to recognise that ecological correlates may have only indirect significance: only 7% DSH patients themselves live in overcrowded conditions.

Early parental separation: 34% men, 26% women.
Previous criminal record: 30% men, 6% women.
Unemployment: clear association among men in Edinburgh during the period 1968–1982. The incidence in men was more than ten times higher in the unemployed than among the employed. As the rate of unemployment rose in Oxford during 1979–1982, it was closely paralleled by increase in the proportion of male DSH patients who were unemployed. There was, however, no clear relationship between overall male DSH rates and rate of unemployment, although there was a clear positive link with duration of unemployment. Explanation of these statistical associates needs to be cautious, and any causal link may be indirect.

64% some major precipitating event.
50% interpersonal upset.
Less commonly, anxiety over work or finance, illness, housing,
bereavement, antisocial behaviour.
25% no upset admitted.

45% do not have close friend, 35% feel personally isolated at all times.

Major psychotic illness	14% males	11% females
Chronic alcohol abuse	25%	7%
Alcohol intake within 6 hours	55%	25%
Reactive depression	39%	59%
Personality disorder	42%	22%
Organic psychosis	17%	6%

MOTIVATION AND CAUSES

	Male(%)	Female(%)
At the time of DSH wish to die	46	34
By the next day regret not dying	17	10
Evidence of serious intent to die	10	10

The majority are impulsive acts in relation to upsetting event which
precipitates depression in someone who is vulnerable, but only a
small minority mentally ill. Facilitated by recent intake of alcohol.
    Reasons given for the episode:
    — seek help
    — escape from situation
    — relief from state of mind
    — attempt to influence someone.
    Ordeal character: gamble between life and death
    Appeal or communicational effect: 18% are aware of one or more
similar episode in first degree relative.
    Self laceration may have obsessive-compulsive character in
some, or hysterical change in state of consciousness with
anaesthesia of mortified part. Can be a difficult problem in prisons or
other institutions in which freedom of movement limited. Secondary
gain may be important, often in impulsive aggressive personality.
    Alcohol problems most marked in middle aged men and in those
living in city centres.
    Inappropriate prescription of psychotropic drugs also important.

COMPARISON BETWEEN SUICIDE AND NON-FATAL DELIBERATE SELF HARM (DSH)

Suicide	DSH
Overall rates fell in 1960's.	Marked increase in rates in 1960's.
Rates increase with age.	Rates fall as age increases.
Rare in children.	Rare in children.
More common in males.	More common in females.
Drug poisoning most common cause but physical violence not infrequent.	Massive preponderance of drug overdosage.
	Only minority have conscious idea of suicide. 1% commit suicide in following year (10% in long term), only 10% are 'failed suicides'.

PREDICTION OF REPETITION

At 0.001 level

Previous episode of DSH, psychiatric treatment or criminal record.

At 0.01 level

Social Class IV or V, separated, episode not precipitated by upset, drug dependence, early separation (before 15 years) from mother.

ASSESSMENT AFTER DSH FOR HIGH RISK SUICIDE OR REPEAT NFDSH

Age and sex. Males age 35 years or older.

Act of DSH. Severe, especially extensive laceration, precaution to avoid discovery, premeditated 24 hours or more, no obvious precipitating factors, conscious suicide intent.

Preceding symptoms. Persistent depression, self blame, anger, resentment, impulsive behaviour, psychosis, serious alcohol or drug problem, serious physical discord, persistent somatic symptoms.

Social. Recurrent crises, lack support, separated, live alone, in city centre.

Personal. Suicide in first degree relative, separated from parents for six months or more before age 15 years, episode of DSH in previous three months, previous psychiatric treatment.

Status after episode. Persistent depression, anger, resentment, uncooperative, continuing suicidal ideas, unresolved or worsening situation.

TREATMENT AND PREVENTION

The Hill Report in 1968 recommended that all cases of deliberate self harm should be referred to designated Treatment Centres in District General Hospitals and seen by psychiatrists.
Implementation of this advice has been very incomplete and considerable variation exists in the way these patients are treated.

It has been demonstrated that in certain circumstances, medical practitioners (other than psychiatrists), nurses and social workers can be as effective as psychiatrists in the initial psychosocial evaluation of patients admitted to hospital following DSH.
Delegation of psychiatric responsibility should however only occur in a well organised scheme where prompt psychiatric advice is readily available and good communication exists between all staff involved, who also obtain adequate preliminary training in assessment of suicide and DSH risk.
Recent DHSS guidelines on the management of deliberate self harm (DHSS 1984). These may be summarised as follows:

1. The initial priority should be the management of the physical condition, but subsequent evaluation of the psychiatric and social state is essential in every case. Medical staff other than psychiatrists may, where appropriate, carry out initial assessment and decide the need for psychiatric referral. In some instances other professional workers such as social worker, nurse or clinical psychologist may also do so.
2. Certain patients may be managed at home by general practitioners.
3. Patients discharged from accident and emergency departments should have full psychosocial assessment.
4. Each hospital should have a clear code of practice on the management of deliberate self harm. A standing multidisciplinary committee is recommended.
5. Minimal standards of care should be made clear.
6. All children under 12 who are referred because of deliberate self harm should be admitted as in-patients, preferably to a paediatric ward. This is also desirable for children aged 12–16.
7. Staff should be aware that apparently minor physical risk does not necessarily mean low risk of repetition.
8. Designation of special beds or provision of a poison treatment centre is desirable.
9. Immediate availability of psychiatric advice at all times is essential.
10. Specialist social workers, nurses and clinical psychologists might undertake assessment of some cases and undertake after-care.
11. Teaching on deliberate self harm should be arranged regularly for all relevant staff groups.

Even though 50–55% of cases are referred to psychiatric clinics, they show a high default rate.

No effective way of reducing repetition rate yet demonstrated, either using psychiatric or social work techniques.

'First ever' cases respond best.

Patients show variety of attitudes to help: 36% prefer GP, 23% are recurrent psychiatric attenders, 41% do not readily seek help from anyone.

> Problem orientated approach involves:
> Identification of problem
> Establishment of goals
> Clarification of steps to achieve goals
> Choice of tasks
> Review of progress
> Modification of attitudes
> Facilitation of communication
> Contracting
> Providing information (about DSH).
> Psychotherapy often involves:
> > long term support setting limits
> > treatment of significant depression
> > use of conjoint situation

Primary prevention may be most fruitful approach (early intervention, provision of adequate support especially when psychotropic drugs prescribed for persons with life difficulties).

FURTHER READING

DHSS (1984) *The Management of Deliberate Self Harm*. Health Notice 84(25).
Hawton, K. & Catalan, J. (1987) *Attempted Suicide*. 2nd ed. Oxford: Oxford University Press.
Kreitman, N. (Ed.) (1977) *Parasuicide*. Chichester: John Wiley.
Morgan, H. G. (1979) *Death Wishes*? Chichester: John Wiley.

C. MENTAL HEALTH SERVICES

PREVALENCE OF MENTAL DISORDER

National Morbidity Survey 1970–1971. Office of Population Census and Surveys.

Based on 53 general practices in England and Wales.

1 in 14 males ⎱ consult a general practitioner because
1 in 7 females ⎰ of mental illness per year.

Of these 12% referred to specialist services.

Anxiety state   20 male, 47 female ⎱
Depressive neurosis 15 male, 47 female ⎰ per 1000 attended GP.
Affective psychosis 1 in 280.
Schizophrenic psychosis 1 in 300.

PATTERN OF PSYCHIATRIC SERVICES

Since 1950s progressive increase in emphasis on community based facilities as opposed to those in large psychiatric hospitals.
Uncertainty regarding the future role of mental hospitals.
Progressive fall in numbers of patients requiring long term hospital care.

THE HEALTH DISTRICT	Population approximately 250 000	
Mental Health Service Provision (Adults)	Beds per 100 000	Day places
Psychiatric units in district		
general hospital	50	65
Elderly severely mentally infirm	30–40	25–40
New long stay patients	31	
Peripheral day hospital		30
Local Authority Provision (Adults)		
Hostels in community	4–6	
Long stay accommodation	15–24	
Day centre		60

Increasing emphasis on voluntary agencies in providing comprehensive service.

The District General Hospital (DGH) Psychiatric Unit is intended as the centre of specialist psychiatric treatment for adults, including compulsorily detained patients.

The majority will be ambulant, stay for a few weeks only.

Rather more than half day places used by in-patients.

The Elderly Mentally Infirm (EMI) would be treated separately, or together with other psychiatric patients in DGH unit.

A few (ESMI) will need continuing care usually because of dementia: preferably in small community hospitals (2.5–3.0 per 1000 age 65+).

Joint assessment unit with geriatricians (e.g. 10–20 beds for this purpose in each health district).

As population gets older the required facilities for the elderly will increase considerably in the next few decades. The population in the year 2000 compared with the present will be: total: 104%; 64–75 years: 90%; 75 years and over: 128%.

Long term care of chronic mental illness

In 1971, of patients in mental illness hospital, 73% had been there more than one year, 41% more than ten years.

Excluding dementia, other forms of chronic mental illness still develop.

The new long stay patients who stay in hospital 1–3 years.
Sample evaluated by Mann and Cree.
One third need continuous medical/nursing supervision.
Remainder need sheltered environment in community.
0.17 per 1000 beds required in each health district.
Ideal placement uncertain. DGH units not most suitable. Hostel near hospital campus may be best.

Chronic organic brain damage
Placements a problem especially when behaviour disorder complicates it.

Services for children
Continued expansion of hospital services a high priority.
   Prime emphasis will need to be on early intervention in home, school, health centre and other community bases.
   Close collaboration between many agencies required and involvement of whole families as well as other key personnel.

Services for adolescents
Evidence that psychiatric morbidity is higher than in adults, yet adolescents reluctant to seek help.
Special needs must be taken into account.
Informal walk-in clinics useful.
Voluntary agencies invaluable in providing this approach.

FUTURE OF THE MENTAL HOSPITAL

Aim at a period of transition rather than dissolution.
Emphasis increasingly towards day hospital and other community care.
The DGH psychiatric unit may become complete service.
In other districts, the mental hospital will continue to have supportive role.
Need to avoid two-tier system in which mental hospital remains under-privileged.
Need to define type of patient appropriate for mental hospital of the future: these might include EMI, new long stay and old long stay, special units.
Joint planning between Health Authorities and Social Services crucial.

COMMUNITY CARE

Long standing support for the policy of community care (DHSS 1976)

Aims
Keep disabled people in own homes, or homelike environment, for as long as possible rather than in large institutions.
Preserve consumers' right to choose services and clothing, meals, bedtimes, friends and social activities.

Implementation
This has been unsatisfactory. Enormous variability of community services and funding from one area to another. Funding inflexible, uncoordinated, and involvement of multiple organisations leads to confusion of responsibility. Health and social services are separate, and frequently have differing priorities.

Mental illness
Places in psychiatric hospitals reduced by 25 000 during 1974–84, yet residential places provided by local authorities, private and voluntary sectors increased by only 9000. Those remaining in hospital have severe disabilities, and it becomes progressively more difficult to find alternative care for them. Recent survey of Salvation Army hostels in central London reveals that 35% of residents have chronic schizophrenia, often not in contact with psychiatric services.

Mental handicap
In 1971 the DHSS envisaged that more than 50% of care provision should be in ordinary houses and flats. By 1985 only 21% of mentally handicapped patients were being cared for in this way.

The elderly
There will be an increase of 50% in numbers of persons over 85 years of age in Britain between now and the end of the century. Remarkable growth of private nursing homes but the demand on services will clearly be enormous.

The four components of good community care (King's Fund 1986 and 1987)
Clear values and principles about what community care services are trying to achieve.
The views of the recipients of services must be considered.
Professional knowledge and techniques of treatment and care play a valuable role.
Access to all the usual community services should be ensured.

Six features which foster innovation (Audit Commission 1986)
The existence of strong and committed local champions of change.
Focus on action and achievement rather than maintaining the status quo.

Local integrated services with collaboration between statutory and voluntary agencies.

Focus on the local neighbourhood.

Multi-disciplinary team approach.

Partnership between strategy and voluntary agencies.

FURTHER READING

The Audit Commission (1986) *Making a Reality of Community Care*. London: HMSO.

DHSS (1971) *Better Services for the Mentally Handicapped*. London: HMSO.

DHSS (1986) *Priorities for Health and Personal Social Services in England*. London: HMSO.

King's Fund (1987) *Facilitating Innovation in Community Care*. London.

Murphy, E. (1987) Community care I: problems. *Brit. Med. J.*, **295**, 1505–1508.

Murphy, E. (1988) Community care II: possible solutions. *Brit. Med. J.*, **296**, 6–8.

PROVISION OF SECURITY

Patient should only be placed in conditions of special security when strictly necessary and no alternatives possible.

Regional security units

Recommended by Butler Committee and DHSS.

Care of patients who need greater supervision than the open-door system can provide, yet do not require security in one of the special hospitals.

Butler Committee expressed concern at lack of appropriate local provision for this type of patient: pointed out that many offenders are sent to prison instead of hospital as a result. About one quarter of prisoners have significant mental disturbance.

To be financed from central government funds, recent arrangements to provide revenue as well as capital support.

Selection of patients under discussion.

Variety of regimes: some provide locked door security, others use open door policy with high staff/patient ratio.

Local forensic psychiatric service essential to provide early assessment and constant support in parallel with regional security unit.

Special hospital provision of extra security for mentally-disturbed patients and offenders 20/million general population or a total nationally of about 2000 beds.

FURTHER READING

DHSS (1975) *Better Services for the Mentally Ill*. London: HMSO.
DHSS/Home Office (1975) *Report of the Committee on Mentally Abnormal Offenders*. London: HMSO.
Early, D. F. & Nicholas M. (1977) Dissolution of the mental hospitals. *Brit. J. Psychiat.*, **130**, 117–122.
Mann & Cree, W. (1975) The 'new long stay' in mental hospitals. *Brit. J. Hosp. Med.*, July, 56–63.

D. TERMINATION OF PREGNANCY

THE ABORTION ACT 1967

Termination permissible if
a) continuation of pregnancy would involve risk to the life of the pregnant woman, or of injury to her physical and mental health or that of any existing children of her family, greater than if the pregnancy was terminated.
b) there is a substantial risk that if the child was born, if would suffer from such physical or mental abnormality as to be seriously handicapped.

The pregnant woman's actual or reasonably foreseeable environment can be taken into account in reaching a decision.

ASSESSMENT PROBLEMS

Guilt and regret after termination is most common in those women who show the most severe psychiatric disturbance at the time abortion is requested.

In a series of women refused abortion, 73% subsequently satisfied with decision.

In women who received abortions 25% self reproachful.

Remember that termination of pregnancy is not without risks (especially infection and haemorrhage) mortality 0.6 per 1000.

Risks much increased after 12 weeks gestation.

PSYCHIATRIC INDICATIONS FOR TERMINATION

In the mother
1. History of recurrent puerperal psychosis or of one intractible puerperal illness especially if schizophrenic in type: high risk of recurrence with further pregnancy.
2. Acute emotional upset with suicide risk. 20% threaten suicide though it is rare in women refused abortion. Unwise to ignore, assess carefully, preferably in hospital, especially when severe depressive symptoms such as morbid guilt are present or recurrent self injury under stress.

3. Chronic mental illness, especially disabling schizophrenic psychosis.
4. Mental handicap. Poor standard of care of existing children, especially when a further child might mean family breakdown.

In the child
Rubella in first 20 weeks of pregnancy.
Maternal smallpox, vaccination, exposure to cytotoxic drugs or X-rays. (30 rads or more to pelvis within first trimester).
Familial illness (pheylketonuria, galactosaemia, haemophilia, Christmas disease).
Chromosomal defects: mongolism (1 in 70 chance of a second mongol child occurring in a family with one child already affected: increased risk in older mothers).

FURTHER READING

Granville-Grossman, K. (1971) *Recent Advances in Clinical Psychiatry-1* pp. 266–280. Edinburgh: Churchill Livingstone.

E. INFANTILE AUTISM AND OTHER CHILD PSYCHOSES

SCHIZOPHRENIA

Occurs most often during adolescence: onset may be as early as 7 years of age.
Symptomatology identical with that in adults. 10% parents schizophrenic.
Excess of boys.
Childhood precursors of adult schizophrenia include: poor academic attainment, social isolation, personality oddities, I.Q. slightly below average.

DISINTEGRATIVE PSYCHOSIS

Normal up to 3rd and 4th year, when profound regression and behaviour disintegration occurs. Loss of speech, language, social skills, interest in objects, development of stereotypes and mannerisms.
   Occasionally follows measles, encephalitis or similar illness but usually no clear precipitating illness.

MANIC DEPRESSIVE PSYCHOSIS

Rare.

INFANTILE AUTISM

First described by Kanner in 1943. Generally regarded as being quite
distinct from schizophrenia (occurs in infancy with low incidence of
family schizophrenia, evidence of cerebral dysfunction, low I.Q., and
has distinctive symptom pattern. Less likely to follow remitting
pattern and rarely develop delusions and hallucinations in
adulthood).

Prevalence
4 per 10 000 children have psychosis. Half of these comprise the
specific syndrome of autism.

Symptoms and diagnostic criteria
Three kinds:
a) profound general failure to develop social and individual
   relationships.
b) language retardation (impaired comprehension, echolalia,
   pronominal reversal).
c) ritualistic compulsive phenomena (insistence on sameness)
   stereotyped, repetitive movement (especially hand and finger
   mannerisms).
   short attention span, self injury, delayed bowel control.
Onset before 30 months. In 80% development has clearly been
abnormal from birth.
I.Q. probably below average. 75% score in retarded range in spite of
good motivation.
   May be good rote memory and visuospatial function and these
together with absence of physical stigmata, can be misleading in I.Q.
assessment.
   Fundamental defect may be a cognitive disorder involving
language and central coding processes.
   Pattern of scores on I.Q. tests different from those of mentally
retarded children. Prognosis worse when I.Q. low.

Impaired social relationships
Lack of attachment behaviour and relative failure of bonding most
marked in first five years (do not follow parents around the house,
do not turn to them for comfort, nor distinguish between people).
   Unusual use of eye to eye gaze.
   Lack of cooperative group play, failure to make friendships, lack of
empathy.
   Says or does socially inappropriate things: gaucheness in later
years prevents close relationships.

Language and other skills
Impaired imitation or meaningful use of objects and lack of imaginative play.

Babble speech abnormal (usually present in 2 year old).

Impaired comprehension of spoken language especially if it involves 2 or more ideas.

Lack gesture and mime.

Pronominal reversal ('you' instead of 'I') and echolalia. Unusual use of words and metaphors.

Talks less than normal.

In later years speech may lack cadence and inflexion and may seem pedantic and formal.

Insistence on sameness
Rigid, limited play patterns, lacking imagination.

Resist change in environment.

Intense attachment to toys and other objects.

Unusual preoccupation which excludes others (bus routes, train timetables, patterns, colours, numbers).

Ask stereotyped questions which require fixed answers.

Obsessional symptoms may develop later.

Variety of other behaviour
Feeding difficulties in infancy, stereotypies of hands, spinning of whole body or objects, self injury.

Causes
Likely to be a behavioural syndrome without a single cause but with common biological causation: may include several distinct syndromes.

Some type of cognitive deficit likely (use of language as above).

Organic brain defect suggested in retarded autistics because 28% of these later develop epilepsy in adolescence.

Radiological studies suggest enlargement of temporal horn: possible medial temporal lobe pathology.

Increased incidence of non-specific EEG abnormalities.

Cytogenetic and biochemical: no consistent abnormality demonstrated.

Concordance in twins high in those without evidence of organic brain dysfunction.

Autism may be common in hypsarrhythmia, mental retardation and sensory deficit secondary to congenital rubella.

Treatment
Few recover completely but treatment can in many lead to
improvement and social adjustment.
Recent trend away from insight directed psychotherapy with child
towards:
— facilitating normal social and linguistic development in spite of
  congenital defect.
— avoidance of secondary handicaps.
— emphasis on treating pre-school child.
— helping total family.
— special educational provision (systematic rather than
  permissive approach probably better. Poor response
  associated with low I.Q.).
— drugs used symptomatically, e.g. major tranquillisers for
  behaviour control.
— behavioural techniques can be useful (operant or desensitation
  useful in reducing deviant disruptive behaviour).

PROGNOSIS

60% remain severely handicapped and totally unable to lead
independent life.
16% make good social adjustment and obtain a job (most remain
eccentric with poor relationships).
24% intermediate outcome.
28% develop epilepsy (closely related to low I.Q.).

Indicators of poor outcome
Low I.Q. the most important, though a substantial proportion of
intelligent autistic children do not do well.
Failure to acquire language by 5 years.
Severe behaviour disturbance in early childhood.
Disrupted disharmonious home.

FURTHER READING

Kolvin, I & Macmillan, A (1976) Child psychiatry. In *Recent Advances in
Clinical Psychiatry-2*. ed. K. Granville-Grossman. Edinburgh: Churchill
Livingstone.
Rutter, M. (1977) Infantile autism and other child psychoses. In *Child
Psychiatry*. ed. Rutter & Hersov. Oxford: Blackwell Scientific.

F. ENURESIS

DEFINITION

Difficult to select point at which this becomes abnormal because
prevalence curve shows smooth decline with increasing age.

Poussaint and Ditman: Nocturnal enuresis may be defined as nocturnal bedwetting in a child in whom the act of voiding otherwise occurs in the normal way.

This does not cover diurnal enuresis in which child is wet day and night.

Werry: Wetting in the school age period. This definition is useful because prevalence low at this age, spontaneous remission low, and child likely to be concerned at it.

TYPES

Primary (or continuous): never been dry.
Secondary (or onset): dry for at least a year then wet again.

EPIDEMIOLOGY

Prevalence at 5 years 17% (N.E. England), 10% (Stockholm), 32% Negroes in Baltimore.

Associated with social handicap in family.
Prevalence higher in boys than girls.

CAUSAL THEORIES

Physical or physiological

Sensitive period for emergence of dryness. Most children establish this between 18 and 54 months. Any interference with bladder control during this sensitive period might mean that child will be without control for a number of years.

Genetic. MZ twins twice as concordant as DZ. Well known high familial incidence may be related to family custom.

Functional bladder capacity (as opposed to structural capacity). Failure of ability to hold urine for increasing periods in the day with extension into sleeping state.

Deep sleep pattern. Little evidence for this, either EEG or otherwise.

Developmental delay. Consistent with tendency to spontaneous remission with increasing age, higher incidence in low birth weight children, poorer physical growth in enuretics, excess of boys (in common with other developmental disorders).

Physical factors. Urinary infection (in 10% of girls who wet nightly). Little consistent association with urinary tract defects.

Learning theory explanations

Nocturnal continence probably achieved by complementary action of neurophysiological maturity and learning processes.

Poor social conditions and training. Low I.Q. may impair learning.

Psychodynamic
Increased incidence of psychological disturbance in enuretics especially in girls, but 70% are without psychiatric difficulties.

No association of enuresis with any specific syndrome.

Anxiety provoked by stress may lead to bladder irritability and hence impede learnt bladder control in predisposed children.

No specificity of stress demonstrated.

Need to distinguish early adverse factors from later perpetuating ones: Douglas found excess of stress at age 3 years in enuretics.

VARIETIES OF ENURESIS

Newcastle. Primary type: primarily biological basis. Secondary type: psychogenic.

Maudsley. Nocturnal (more common in boys), mainly developmental and biological. Diurnal (more common in girls) associated with behaviour disorder.

TREATMENT

Guidance for parents, helping stressed families.
Minimise over-critical or punishing parental attitudes.
Encourage success.
Lifting 2–3 hours after going to bed.
Fluid restriction in evenings.
Bell and pad technique may help some: effects more persistent than antidepressants.
Psychotherapy effective only when there is good evidence of associated emotional disorder.
Antidepressant medication e.g. Imipramine. May act by anticholinegic effect, though long term follow up suggests that relapse likely as soon as it is stopped. Potentially toxic and if no response in 4 weeks, discontinue.
Chlordiazepoxide when anxiety high.
Better response to drugs:
— secondary enuresis
— other milestones achieved normally
— no family history of enuresis.

FURTHER READING

Kolvin, I. & Macmillan, A. (1976) Child psychiatry. In *Recent Advances in Clinical Psychiatry–2*. ed. Granville-Grossman, K. Edinburgh: Churchill Livingstone.

G. THE PSYCHIATRY OF ADOLESCENCE

Exact age range ill-defined: 12–19 year olds comprise 11.5% of population (5.3 million). The major experience during adolescence is one of transition.

Puberty marks the onset of adolescence. In girls there is a critical weight at which the pubertal sequence is triggered: to be precise this is when body fat increases to 22% of total body weight (Frisch & Revelle 1971). During the last 150 years the menarche has occurred progressively earlier by 4 months per decade in Western Europe.

Physical changes

In boys growth spurt begins at 13 years (maximum at 14).

In girls growth spurt begins at 10–11 years (maximum at 11–12).

Considerable individual variation. Sexual maturation closely linked, tends to occur 18–24 months later in boys. Menarche occurs after the peak velocity of growth spurt.

Psychological changes

Maturation of logical reasoning and ability to look at problems from a variety of perspectives utilising abstract concepts. Major changes in the way the world is conceptualised. Piaget: Change from concrete operational to abstract logic and reasoning.

Strives towards independence, frequently associated with ambivalence and rejection of adult values.

Intense examination of capabilities and goals (identity crisis — Erikson).

Adolescence has only recently become a prolonged intermediate period of education and peer group activities between childhood and adult life.

Social changes

Altered expectation from others (academic, job).

Expectation of conformity with peer group and conflict with parents.

COMMON SYMPTOMS

Rutter (Isle of Wight study of 14 year olds) showed that minor conflicts with parents were common. Severe family conflict always needs assessment in case intervention may help.

21% of 14 year olds were found to have psychiatric disorder but in only 10% was this obvious to adults.

Alienation from parents more frequent in those with psychiatric disorder. Leslie (industrial town, N. England) 12–16 year olds: 6% boys, 3% girls severe handicapping psychiatric disorder, 15% boys, 11% girls moderate disorder.

Anxiety and depressive feelings occur in about half of normal adolescents. May be marked lability of mood.

May over-react to stress and appear egocentric in attitude. Incur conflict with parents who see them as selfish and inconsiderate.

SYNDROMES IN ADOLESCENCE

Conduct disorder

A persistent picture of antisocial symptoms usually combined with abnormal interpersonal relationships.

More common in boys, especially from unstable, unhappy families. Often associated with reading difficulties.

Promiscuity and extra-marital pregnancy in girls.

Testing-out common: push others to the limit of tolerance or further.

Neurosis

Anxiety, phobias, depression.

Preoccupation with relationship difficulties and sexual/bodily functions.

School refusal.

Anorexia nervosa.

Gilles de la Tourette syndrome. Multiple motor and vocal tics, the former beginning in childhood, the latter developing later, most commonly at around 13 years. A rare condition, three to four times more common in males. The vocal tics include grunting, snarling, coprolalia (uttering obscenities), echolalia, jumping, dancing. Uncertain whether functional or organic factors paramount in aetiology. Haloperidol or pimozide said to be useful in treatment, but prognosis is guarded.

Suicide

Rare in adolescence but more common than in children.
? more common in adolescents of high I.Q. and above average stature.

Attempted suicide

7–10% of referrals to child psychiatric clinics are for the threatened or attempted suicide (Shaffer).

Psychosis

Insidious onset of schizophrenia during adolescence may denote poor prognosis.

Drugs and alcohol abuse

Experimentation may begin in adolescence.

TREATMENT

Referral rates tend to be low even though psychiatric disorders slightly more common than in adults.

? related to reluctance to seek help.

Specialist approach geared to adolescents' needs is justified: facilities for younger ones need to be different from those for older ones.

4 beds per 100 000 required for younger adolescents.

Need to work with entire family (e.g. setting goals).

Adolescent units need close links with schools and the community especially voluntary agencies.

Variety of approaches being explored.

Family therapy particularly useful in adolescence:
— brings all relevant information into the open.
— other family members need help when adolescent member has problems.
— prevents obstructive resistance from relatives.
— dilutes adolescent's hostility to therapist.
— helps family to tolerate adolescent.
— may prevent unnecessary hospital admission.

FURTHER READING

Brugger, P. & Davies, G. (1977) Family therapy in adolescent psychiatry. *Brit. J. Psychiat.*, **131**, 433–447.

DHSS (1975) *Better Services for the Mentally Ill: Adolescents.* pp. 58–61. London: HMSO.

DHSS (1986) *Bridges over Troubled Waters.* A report from the NHS Health Advisory Service on Services for Disturbed Adolescents.

Wolkind, S. N. & Coleman, J. C. (1976) The psychiatry of adolescence. *Brit. J. Hosp. Med.*, June **15**, 575–582.

H. NON-ACCIDENTAL INJURY IN CHILDREN

Kempe in 1962 coined the term 'battered baby'.

CAUSES

A description of behaviour which may be due to a variety of causes.

May be related to:
— a wish to eliminate an encumbrance.
— a wish to relieve suffering.
— disordered thinking in mentally ill parent.
— displacement of anger, frustration, or retaliation.
— a problem in the child itself.

INCIDENCE

Major injury: 1 in 1000 children under 4 years per annum England and Wales.

About 2–4% of children in subnormality hospitals are brain damaged because of assault, usually by violent shaking or battering.

About 25% of severely attacked children are intellectually damaged as a result.

60% chance of repetition. 19% of sibs are 'battered'.

CLINICAL FEATURES

Found in all social classes.

Parents may vary greatly in intelligence, attractiveness, mental stability, personality and apparent efficiency in running the home. They may themselves have suffered abuse.

In the child
Evidence of successive injuries especially bruises of different ages. Bizarre injuries.

All fractures in children up to 2 years of age should be viewed with suspicion.

Non-accidental poisoning with drugs: may cause behavioural changes which are sometimes bizarre: parents may abuse drugs themselves.

May be fearful towards adults or show over-anxious concern for the parents' welfare. Often unhappy.

In the parents
May be evasive, provide contradictory information, lack warmth towards child, lack confidence in handling it, or express overt criticism e.g. its refusal to be comforted, or its excessive crying.

FACTORS PREVENTING EARLY DIAGNOSIS

Incomplete and misinterpreted facts
Ignorance of what to look for and ask, shortage of time, fear of arousing anger or litigation, wish to maintain confidentially, being deceived by parents who may be plausible and misleading.

Available but uncollected information
Mobility of family, deliberate change of doctor or hospital to conceal successive assaults, inaccurate identification of the child concerned, lack of standardised records, failure to make one person responsible for collation of information (key worker).

Unavailable information

Concealment in privacy of home (neighbour may be useful informant): the tradition of protecting the client may obscure the needs of the child.

PREVENTION AND TREATMENT

Good and immediate communication between different branches of caring services essential.

Regional and Area Review Committees set up for this purpose.

Case registers a further important development.

When a suspect case arises, a conference of all helping persons is called and further action agreed by group decision. Key worker nominated as integrator.

If child at immediate risk, may need urgent admission to hospital for assessment and treatment. Occasionally when child in danger and parents object, it may be necessary to remove it compulsorily and urgently under a Place of Safety order. This may lead on to a care order or warding of the child.

FURTHER READING

Rogers, D. et al. (1976) Non-accidental poisoning: an extended syndrome of child abuse. *Brit. Med. J.*, **1**, 793–796.

Working Party of the Royal College of Psychiatrists (1977) *Brit. J. Psychiat.*, **131**, 366–380.

I. THE DIAGNOSIS OF CHILD SEXUAL ABUSE

Kempe in 1979 commented on the serious plight of sexually abused children.

Recent recognition that inconsistent evidence from a child, even withdrawal of statement, may be due to 'accommodation' to a family demand to maintain secrecy. Previously regarded as evidence of fantasy on the part of the child.

More prevalent than previously thought. Up to 20% of girls and 10% of boys experience some form of inappropriate sexual contact in childhood. Accompanied by sense of victimisation and traumatisation that may be long lasting. Doubling of annual referral rate to one special diagnostic service each year during a recent five year period. Uniform rates in 5–16 year olds, significant number of under fives.

DEFINITION (DHSS 1986 Draft Guidelines)

The involvement of dependent developmentally immature children and young people in activities which they cannot fully comprehend, to which they cannot give informed consent, and which violate the social taboos of the culture and are against the Law.

Includes:
— incest. Sexual intercourse between close relatives within a defined relationship who cannot marry. The concept has been extended to include step relations and other relatives/friends who are not permanent residents of the family. Sexual contact of a deviant kind is also included.
— child pornography. The arranging or photographing of any material involving children or young people in sexual acts.
— child prostitution. Involving children in sexual acts for profit.

DIAGNOSIS

Problems inherent in having to depend upon evidence from children, often not corroborated by the implicated adult.

CIBA foundation working party recommends the following guidelines:
— Adequate sharing of confidential information with others who are assisting the doctor in his professional relationship with the patient; when a very serious crime is involved this may override a doctor's duty to maintain confidence.
— Case conferences are vital, in parallel with individual interviews with the child, relatives and the family group. Videotape recordings useful.
— the child's safety is paramount.
— sharing of information is on a 'need to know' basis.
— punitive attitude is counterproductive. Most sexual abuse offenders within the family are not dangerous criminals.

PHYSICAL CONSEQUENCES

Genital, anal damage, ruptured hymen, enlargement of vaginal or anal opening.
Infection (may be of sexually transmitted type)
Pregnancy
Other forms of physical abuse.

PSYCHOLOGICAL CONSEQUENCES

Emotional upset (depression, anxiety), irritability, insomnia
Regressive patterns of behaviour, school failure
Psychosomatic symptoms
Sexualised behaviour: suggestive of an unusual degree of awareness
In adolescents: deliberate self harm, running away, promiscuity, sexual abuse of younger children.

FACTORS ASSOCIATED WITH CHILD SEXUAL ABUSE

Motivational

Confusion of family roles, parental arrested emotional development
Sexual abuse of parents in childhood
Poor sexual adjustment of parents/adults.

Reduced inhibition

Alcohol or drug abuse
Psychotic illness
Low intelligence with poor boundaries in family
Impulse disorders
Absence of protective parent
Child handicapped physically or intellectually.

Family patterns

High secrecy, absence of conflict, intense fears of separation
High levels of conflict, physical violence, neglect.

FURTHER READING

Bentovim, A. (1987) Diagnosis of child sexual abuse. *Bulletin of the Royal College of Psychiatrists*, **11**, 295–299.
Bentovim, A., Elton, A., Hildebrand, J., Tranter, M. & Vizard, E. (1987) *Sexual Abuse in the Family*. Bristol: John Wright.
Ciba Foundation (1984) *Sexual Abuse in the Family*. London: Tavistock.
DHSS (1988) Diagnosis of Child Sexual Abuse. HMSO.
DHSS (1988) Working together. HMSO.

J. MANAGEMENT OF THE VIOLENT PATIENT

Each hospital should have a clear written policy.

All staff must accept responsibility to intervene in any situation where a person may suffer injury: adequate training of medical and nursing staff essential.

Prevention in ward community needs full cooperation between medical and nursing personnel.

The consultant or his deputy should be available at the earliest opportunity following a violent incident for full evaluation and appropriate management.

Potentially violent individuals should only be admitted to wards that have sufficient staff (1:1 recommended by RC Psychiatrists and COHSE).

Avoid excess concentration of difficult patients in one ward especially when it has inadequate facilities.

Emphasis should be on prevention: maintain good ward atmosphere, adequate staff communications and morale. COHSE critical of medical staff attitudes.

Avoid unduly restrictive regime, ensure adequate occupational therapy, preferably away from the ward for part of each day for special group activity.

Note premonitory signs (know patients well).

The violent episode
Establish diagnosis (e.g. alcohol withdrawal states, epileptic episodes).
Staff remain calm and non-critical.
Avoid physical confrontation if possible. Talk and listen to patient.
Need sufficient staff to control outburst without leading to injury.
If restraint necessary use minimal degree of force to control violence, aim to calm rather than provoke.
Use clothing rather than direct bodily restraint if possible but may have to hold hair if patient biting. Never press on neck, chest or abdomen.
Remove patient's shoes.
Great care if intramuscular injection given.
Separate for minimal period, with medical agreement.

Report on violent incidents
Ensure that adequate report is made (as a minimal procedure — in ward report, nursing and medical notes).
Time, place.
Factual account.
Action taken.
Names of all involved.
Description of patient's medical state.
Direction of aggression.
Injury and damage done.
   Nursing Officer responsible for further reporting in the hospital. If actual injury serious or damage to property, copy sent to District Health Authority.
   Injured staff may qualify for Industrial Injury Benefit or Criminal Injuries Compensation (advice sought from DHA immediately).

FURTHER READING

The Management of Violent and Potentially Violent Patients in Hospital.
   DHSS HC(76)11. London:HMSO.

K. PSYCHIATRIC ASPECTS OF AIDS
BACKGROUND

Groups at risk
  1. 70% of all reported cases are homosexual or bisexual men with multiple sexual partners
  2. 15–20% are users of illicit intravenous drugs
  3. Haemophiliacs receiving factor VIII concentrate
  4. Children of high risk individuals
  5. Female sexual partners of men with AIDS.

Transmission
Through exchange of body fluids:
— sexual contact
— transfusion of blood or blood products
— use of contaminated syringes
— to newborn from infected mother.

Casual contact rarely if ever a mode of transmission. Risk to health care professionals low, but avoidance of direct exposure to potentially infected body fluids an important precaution.

Detection
Uncertain proportion of individuals with antibodies to the virus will eventually develop the full AIDS syndrome: estimates range from 25 to 50%. Uncertain latency period between infection and AIDS manifestation.

DISEASE MANIFESTATION

Immunosuppression
This leads to Kaposi's sarcoma, lymphoma, opportunistic infections with protozoa and viruses.

Psychiatric and psychosocial

The 'worried well'
Common in high risk groups. Panic attacks, generalised anxiety, obsessive compulsive disorders, hypochondriasis. 'Pseudo Aids Syndrome' may mimic prodromal symptoms.

Psychiatric symptoms
Resemble reaction to terminal cancer. Initial denial followed by anxiety, depression, hypomania, anger at ineffective medical care, public discrimination, suicidal ideas (self destructive behaviour more likely when personality disorder present).
AIDS dementia may follow various forms of CNS involvement, e.g. non-focal encephalopathy, subacute encephalitis, or focal lesions such as multifocal leucoencephalopathy, vascular complications, cerebral lymphomas. AIDS virus has been isolated from brain tissue.

Dementia related to neuronal loss, cerebral atrophy, glial nodules and microfocal demyelination.

The AIDS dementia syndrome begins with depression, blunted affect, impaired memory, poor concentration, social withdrawal. Assessment should include careful evaluation of cognitive function at an early stage. Deterioration occurs rapidly over a matter of months, with disorientation, secondary delusional ideas, and eventually marked global cognitive deficit.

Social and staff reaction
Danger of excessively defensive negative reaction to AIDS patients, especially when staff are poorly informed about the illness. Detailed guidelines on management procedures are essential.

Management of disturbed behaviour a particular hazard for psychiatric staff. Restraint should only be attempted when staff complement is adequate and the risk of personal injury is rendered as low as possible.

Management
Psychotherapeutic support as in any progressive and fatal illness.

Attention to negative attitudes in others which may lead to patient being ostracised. Development of hospice style care. Minor tranquillisers or antidepressant therapy when symptoms indicate.

Careful attention to suicide risk and management of cognitive impairment.

FURTHER READING

Faulstich, M. E. (1985) Psychiatric aspects of AIDS. *Amer. J. Psychiat.*, **144**, 551–556.

Miller, D., Farmer, R. & Carroll, G. (1985) A pseudo-aids syndrome following from fear of AIDS. *Brit. J. Psychiat.*, **146**, 550–551.

Neurology and neurophysiology in relation to psychiatry

PART TWO

Common clinical problems

A. HEADACHE

Structures sensitive to pain include all extracranial tissues, and intracranial tissues such as basal dura and pia mater, venous sinuses, arteries of the circle of Willis, and nerves with sensory afferents. Brain tissue is insensitive to pain.

TYPES

1. Tension

Description: related to scalp muscle contraction; usually generalised; duration hours; throbbing, clamping, stabbing; scalp tender.

   Treatment: reassurance, analgesics, alleviation of anxiety.

2. Migraine

Description: episodic disorder of function of cranial blood vessels, with unilateral or generalised headache. Often accompanied by nausea, may be preceded or accompanied by transient focal neurological symptoms (e.g. hemiplegic, opthalmoplegic and basilar migraine), female preponderance, often familial. Affects at least 20% of population.

   Investigations: if diagnosis is in doubt, skull X-ray, CT scan.

   Treatment of the attack: analgesics. Ergotamine (if no severe vascular disease).

   Prophylaxis: intermittent courses of tranquillisers, particularly if situational stress. May need to stop contraceptive pill. Clonidine (dixarit) 25–150 μg daily. Pizotifen (Sanomigran) 0.5 mg, usually three a day. Migraleve (buclizine, codeine, paracetamol mixture), 2 tabs at night. Methysergide 2–6 mg daily, restricted course only.

3. Migrainous neuralgia (cluster headache)

Description: episodic, severe pain in eye and face, often at night. Associated with conjunctival suffusion, lacrimation. Duration ½–2 hours: repeated over several weeks, interspersed with prolonged periods of freedom.

   Treatment: oral ergotamine 1–2 mg nightly as preventive.

4. Raised intracranial pressure

Description: paroxysmal, throbbing, bilateral occipital or frontal; aggravated by coughing, bending, straining; worse on waking. May be associated with vomiting. Usually but not necessarily papilloedema. May be transient obscurations of vision and/or diplopia due to VI nerve lesion.

Investigations: skull X-ray — erosion of dorsum sellae; copper — beaten appearance of vault and suture diastasis in children. Chest X-ray. Routine blood count. CT scan. May also need further investigation in special unit, e.g. angiography, contrast encephalography, magnetic resonance imaging (MRI).

5. Low intracranial pressure (relatively rare)

Can arise after lumbar puncture, skull fracture, subdural haematoma, or spontaneously. Severe on standing, relieved by lying. There may be meningism, vomiting.

Treatment: of the cause, and if necessary, saline infusion.

6. Infective (e.g. meningitis, encephalitis, abscess, thrombophlebitis)

Description: generalised, constant, may be meningism, focal CNS signs. Fever.

Investigations: blood count, ESR or viscosity. Chest, skull X-rays. Lumbar puncture *providing there is no* papilloedema, and *no* suspicion of local intracranial lesion.

Treatment: appropriate to the organism and/or local cause.

7. Post-traumatic

Description: generalised, variable duration, worse on bending and with alcohol.

Investigations: skull X-ray, EEG, CAT scan if subdural haematoma suspected (progressive intellectual or memory deficit, variable confusion or disorientation, or focal signs).

8. Toxic

e.g. alcohol, carbon monoxide poisoning, oral contraceptives. Usually clear evidence with careful history.

9. Haemorrhage

a. Subarachnoid

Description: sudden very severe headache in an otherwise fit person. Can be precipitated by straining, exertion. Diffuse or occipital. Usually vomiting, may be clouding of consciousness, meningism, and/or focal CNS signs. 10% have fundal haemorrhages.

Investigations: lumbar puncture, unless papilloedema or focal signs. CAT scan. Angiography to locate site of bleed — needs specialist assessment.

b. Intracerebral
Sudden, severe, with altered consciousness; focal signs common.

10. Hypertensive
Not a common association, but may occur. In acute crises can occur with vomiting. Duration few minutes to hours. Associated optic, fundal and cardiac changes.

11. Cervical spondylosis
Occipital, radiating forwards. Duration hours to days. Precipitated by certain positions of head. Can be caused by whiplash injury.
Investigations: X-ray cervical spine.

12. Opthalmologic causes
Anomalies of refraction. Acute glaucoma: often frontal; vomiting, bradycardia, visual impairment.

13. Cranial arteritis
Constant, localised over temporal, facial and/or occipital arteries. Localised tenderness. Maybe focal CNS signs because of involvement of intracranial vessels. Age of onset > 55 years. Danger — loss of vision.
Investigations: blood count, ESR or plasma viscosity. Local biopsy of vessel.
Treatment: urgent. Prednisolone unless specific contraindications.

14. Cause unknown
In approximately 15% of patients referred to one headache clinic no cause could be found.

FURTHER READING
Bickerstaff, E. R. (1975) Migraine and facial pain. *Medicine*, **34**, 2054–2064.

B. FACIAL PAIN

1. LOCAL PATHOLOGY
Affecting teeth, sinuses, ear, nose, throat, as well as orbital cavity and superior orbital fissure.
Description: pain of variable nature and site.
Investigations: clinical examination; X-rays of skull, orbit, sinuses.

2. FACIAL NEURALGIAS

a. Trigeminal neuralgia

Description: age of onset usually more than 60 years (exceptions V nerve tumours and multiple sclerosis — both rare). Unilateral, stereotyped, severe paroxysms of lancinating pain over localised area of face. Recurrent bursts, with periods of freedom. Relapses and remissions. 'Trigger zones', pain precipitated by stimulation of sensitive areas of the face or gums or by speaking, swallowing, chewing.

Usually affects 2nd and 3rd division first, and later 1st division. No abnormal signs unless symptomatic of local nerve lesion.

Treatment: carbamazepine (Tegretol) up to 6 × 200 mg daily, or phenytoin (Epanutin) up to 300 mg daily, or clonazepam (Rivotril) up to 3 × 200 mg daily (carbamazepine usually most effective). Local injection of nerve branches may be needed for unresponsive cases, and very rarely an injection or operation on the ganglion itself.

b. Auriculotemporal neuralgia (rare)

Usually after lesion in parotid gland. Chewing provokes burning pain, local redness of skin, profuse local sweating in preauricular region.

c. Nasociliary neuralgia (rare)

Episodic or prolonged pain in nasal region, inner canthus and eyeball, with local suffusion. Local trigger zones. Exclude local inflammatory causes and occasional associated aneurysm of carotid.

d. Glossopharyngeal neuralgia (rare)

Paroxysms of severe pain, or prolonged. Unilateral affection of tongue, tonsillar area and pharynx. May radiate to the ear. Precipitated by swallowing, moving tongue, talking. Trigger zones in pharynx.

e. Geniculate neuralgia

Lancing pains in preauricular region, ear, palate, maxilla, mastoid area, may be abnormality of taste and excessive salivation. Can occur with herpes of geniculate ganglion and facial palsy (Ramsay-Hunt syndrome) — cutaneous vesicles in the ear and over mastoid area.

f. Neuralgia of other nerves (rare)

Superior laryngeal nerve, with unilateral hypothyroid pain; auricular branch of vagus nerve with suboccipital pain; Sluder's neuralgia — local nasal pain due to lesion of pterygopalatine ganglion.

g. Raeder's paratrigeminal neuralgia
Severe pain in and around one eye, plus Horner's syndrome.
Continuous progressively severe pain, often due to local malignancy
at base of skull.

h. Costen's syndrome
Shooting pain in mandible and temple, triggered only by chewing or
talking.
    Treatment: adjustment of bite by orthodontic procedures.

3. MIGRAINOUS NEURALGIA (see Headache)

4. ATYPICAL FACIAL NEURALGIA

Description: unilateral, diffuse, burning facial pain. Prolonged
duration, occasionally associated with facial flushing. Usually affects
middle-aged females, who may also be depressed. *N.B.* Exclude
local causes e.g. carious teeth, infected sinuses.
    Treatment: extremely difficult, usually defies analgesics,
ergotamine and antidepressants.

5. POST-HERPETIC NEURALGIA

Pain after local herpes zoster infection. Commonly affects 1st
division V nerve. Continuous burning pain. Affects elderly, who may
also become depressed.
    Treatment: local friction. Analgesics. Avoid addictive drugs.

6. CRANIAL ARTERITIS

Granulomatous arteritis affecting elderly. Pain in face, jaw, and/or
mouth. Worse on eating. Headache — see above. Tender over
superficial arteries.
    May be also muscle pain, tenderness and proximal limb girdle
weakness. *N.B.* Visual loss may be sudden and irreversible.
    Diagnostic: temporal artery biopsy. Raised ESR. Serum α_2
globulin increased, albumin reduced.
    Treatment: initial high doses steroids. Maintenance dose 6
months-1 year, dependent on ESR, plasma viscosity.

7. MYOCARDIAL ISCHAEMIA

Pain in lower jaw, neck, often related to exertion.

FURTHER READING

Bickerstaff, E. R. (1975) Migraine and facial pain. *Medicine*, **34**, 2054.

C. INVOLUNTARY MOVEMENTS

1. TREMOR

Rhythmic sinusoidal movement, maximal when:

a) Limb at rest — 'rest tremor'
   Examples: Parkinson's disease, parkinsonism, rarely cerebral tumours, drugs, e.g. reserpine, tetrabenazine, phenothiazines, butyrophenones.

b) Limb outstretched against gravity — 'postural tremor'.
   Examples: physiological, exaggerated physiological in anxiety states, thyrotoxicosis, alcoholism, drugs e.g. tricyclics, bronchodilators, heavy metal poisoning, benign essential (often familial) tremor, cerebellar lesions, Wilson's disease, neurosyphilis.

c) During voluntary movement — 'intention tremor'.
   Examples: cerebellar or brain stem lesions due to multiple sclerosis, spinocerebellar degenerations, tumours or vascular disease.

2. a. CHOREA

Brief, random, irregular, jerky movements of face, tongue, limbs and trunk. May be followed by voluntary movement in same direction to mask the affliction. Walking can be affected (lurching, stopping, dancing-type gait). Limbs may be hypotonic, power is normal, reflexes retained, flexor plantar responses.

Examples: a) Sydenham's chorea — children or young adults, can recur in later pregnancy. May be unilateral — hemichorea.

b) Huntington's chorea — (with dementia). Autosomal dominant inheritance or sporadic. Onset 30–40 years, progressive. Onset in childhood as an akinetic-rigid Parkinsonian syndrome.

c) Chorea can also occur in thyrotoxicosis, systemic lupus erythematosis, polycythemia rubra vera, encephalitis lethargica, or be induced by drugs, e.g. phenytoin.

b. BALLISMUS OR HEMIBALLISMUS

Sudden, wild limb movements, caused by vascular lesion in contralateral subthalamic nucleus, usually slow spontaneous recovery.

3. MYOCLONUS

Brief, shock-like contractions of muscle groups, causing sudden limb movements. Irregular or rhythmic, often repetitive in some muscles.

Seen in:
Idiopathic epilepsy
Progressive myoclonic epilepsy:
— familial
— Lafora body disease
— lipidoses
— spino-cerebellar degenerations.
Metabolic disorders:
— renal failure
— hepatic failure
— respiratory failure
— alcohol and drug withdrawal.
Structural brain disease:
— post-anoxic
— Creutzfeldt-Jakob disease
— subacute sclerosing leuco-encephalitis
— encephalitis lethargica.

4. TICS

Brief repetitive muscle contractions, invariably stereotyped. Can be controlled with effort. Very common in young children, may persist to adulthood in a few subjects. Specific treatment rarely required. May be severe, associated with repetitive swearing in Gilles de la Tourette's syndrome in childhood.

5. TORSION DYSTONIA (athetosis)

Sustained, irregular, semirotatory muscle spasms distorting the body into characteristic postures e.g. torticollis, retrocollis, lordosis, scoliosis, arm extension, foot plantar flexion and inversion.
   Initially with action, later at rest, maybe resulting persistent limb deformity.
a) Symptomatic in:
— cerebral palsy
— Wilson's disease
— Juvenile Huntington's chorea
— Hallevorden-Spatz disease
— encephalitis lethargica.
b) Drugs: phenothiazines, butyrophenones, metcloplramide, diazoxide.
c) Idiopathic dystonia musculorum deformans (onset in children or adults, intellect normal, cause uncertain).
d) Paroxysmal dystonia — paroxysmal choreoathetosis.

6. LOCALISED INVOLUNTARY MOVEMENTS

a) Hemifacial spasm: brief, unilateral, irregular contractions of facial muscles. Most — no cause, but can follow Bell's Palsy, or indicate VII nerve compression.
b) Blepharospasm: affects orbicularis oculi. Usually idiopathic, most commonly in elderly patients. Also symptomatic in Parkinson's disease or torsion dystonia.
c) Spasmodic torticollis: *Idiopathic* — most common. Age 30–50 years, painful neck, resistant to treatment.
Symptomatic — (trauma or infection of cervical spine, cerebellar tumour in children, drugs e.g. phenothiazines).
d) Writer's cramp: specific inability to write, type or play musical instrument. Resistant to most treatments. Minor tranquillisers and retraining may help in a few.
e) Dyskinesias: tardive e.g. facial, often with chorea of digitis and dystonic trunk movements. Complicate phenothiazine and butyrophenone medication.

7. AKATHISIA

Inability to keep lower limbs still: restless shuffling movements. May accompany drug induced parkinsonism in phenothiazine and butyrophenone medication.

FURTHER READING

Marsden, D. (1975) *Medicine*, **35**, 2146–2156.

D. THE PARKINSONIAN SYNDROME

Characterised by degenerative pathological changes affecting the pigmented nuclei of the brain stem. Nerve cells in the substantia nigra, globus pallidus, and corpus striatum show atrophy and loss of pigmentation. In the idiopathic form there may be prominent eosinophilic intracytoplasmic inclusions — Lewy bodies.

CAUSES

A. Idiopathic
Parkinson's disease (Paralysis Agitans)
    60 000–80 000 patients in UK
    Prevalence: 1 in 1000, rising over age of 50 to 1 in 200.

B. Parkinson's syndrome — Parkinsonism
 1. Post-encephalitic, e.g. after epidemic encephalitis lethargica in 1920s but sporadic since.

2. Arteriosclerotic: often unilateral, rigid-akinetic syndrome, tremor less frequent. Age usually above 60 years, other signs of arteriosclerosis, e.g. mental, pseudo-bulbar palsy or other neurological signs.
3. In certain heredo-familial degenerative disorders, e.g. olivoponto-cerebellar atrophy, Wilson's disease, Huntington's chorea (rigid form), Guam Island dementia and parkinsonian complex.
4. Associated with more diffuse organic brain disease:
   a) senile dementia, presenile dementia, e.g. Alzheimer's disease, Creutzfeld-Jakob disease.
   b) post-anoxic, poisoning and drugs, e.g. carbon monoxide, carbon disulphide, sulphur dioxide, butyrophenones, reserpine.
   c) tumour — rare.
   d) polycythaemia.
   e) progressive supranuclear palsy, with paralysis of ocular movements. Sporadic or familial, age 50–70 years. Usually also dementia, rarely pyramidal and cerebellar signs.
   f) post-traumatic — very rare. Occasionally after single severe episode with permanent brain damage, or after recurrent less severe injuries, e.g. boxers.

SYMPTOMS AND SIGNS

1. Akinesia
Inhibition of primary automatic movements. Loss of facial expression, lack of blinking and other associated expressive movements, loss of normal arm swinging when walking. Festinating gait — small shuffling steps, pro and retropulsion.

2. Rigidity
Increased tone of extrapyramidal type:
a) 'lead-pipe', present throughout passive movements of a limb.
b) resting tone increased, and increase in antagonistic muscle tone.
c) cog-wheel phenomenon — stepwise variation in tone with passive alternating movements of pronation/supination or flexion/extension.
d) postural abnormality — bent forwards, knees and elbows flexed. May lead to skeletal deformities.

3. Tremor
Rhythmic, sinusoidal movements of a limb at frequency 4–8 per second. Typically maximal at rest, abolished by voluntary movement, but can persist as action tremor. Increased by emotion, abolished in sleep. Finger tremor — 'pill rolling'.

4. Other physical changes
(*N.B.* normal reflexes, flexor plantar responses if uncomplicated).
Micrographia.
Quiet monotonous voice; poor articulation, word repetition
(echolalia).
Respiratory abnormality (irregular frequency and depth).
Accentuated nasopalpebral reflex — positive glabellar tap sign.
Autonomic symptoms (especially post-encephalitic, seborrhoea,
dribbling, sweating attacks).
Oculogyric crises (post-encephalitic and drug induced). Fixed
upward deviation of eyes for minutes or hours, occasionally also
head tilting.

5. Mental changes
Initially usually none. Later apathy, emotional lability (especially
with supranuclear palsy), depression. Dementia when complicating
brain disease. *N.B.* Acute confusional states, hallucinations, apathy,
lethargy, can be drug induced or herald intercurrent infection.

TREATMENT

Medical

a. Drugs

1. Laevodopa. Originally given alone, now usually in combination
with a selective extracerebral decarboxylase inhibitor. Latter
prevents conversion of dopa to dopamine outside the brain, but fails
to enter brain tissues, so allows increased efficacy of lower dose
within the brain. Reduces side effects. Sinemet 275 (250 mg L dopa,
25 mg carbidopa). Sinemet 110 (L dopa 100 mg, carbidopa 10 mg),
dose: up to 6 × 275. Madopar (100 mg L dopa, 25 mg benserazide),
dose: up to 6 a day.
  Side effects: nausea, vomiting, weight loss, hypotension.
        involuntary movements — dose related.
        psychiatric complications such as confusional state
        (in 25%), but remits with reduced dose.
        contraindicated with monoamine oxidase inhibitors,
        in recent myocardial infarction, and may exacerbate
        glaucoma.

2. Amantadine: (Symmetrel) 100 mg bd or tds. Initially moderately
potent but effect may diminish. Reduce dose slowly to avoid
rebound effects. Side effects — ankle oedema, skin changes,
confusional states.

3. *Anticholinergics*, e.g.   benzhexol (Artane, Pipanol) up to 15 mg
daily.
orphenadrine (Disipal) up to 400 mg daily.
benztropine (Cogentin) up to 6 mg daily —
moderate effect on rigidity, akinesia, less
effect on tremor.

Side effects: dry mouth, blurred vision, constipation, urinary
retention, confusional state.

4. *Bromocriptine* (directly acting dopamine agonist). More
prolonged action than L dopa.

5. *Propranolol.* Can help tremor.

6. *Physiotherapy.* Help with walking and activities of daily living.
Often particularly useful in conjunction with phase of drug induced
improvement.

7. Later in the illness short periods of drug withdrawl — drug
holidays — can help.

Surgical
Stereotactic operation.
   Mechanical, chemical, electrical or cryogenic lesion in globus
pallidus to diminish rigidity, or in posterolateral nucleus of thalamus
to reduce tremor. A rare procedure since advance of L dopa. Rigidity
most likely to be helped, tremor less likely, and akinesia least
amenable.
   Indications: unilateral disease, significant social disability,
unresponsive to full medication.
   Contraindications: previous cerebrovascular accident,
hypertension, marked mental changes, relative contraindications,
age more than 65 years.

FURTHER READING

Mumenthaler, M. (1976) *Neurology*. Chicago: Thieme.

Neurological investigations

1. X-RAYS OF THE SKULL may show:

a) Fractures.
b) Localised or generalised alteration in skull thickness or local defects.
c) Abnormal shape, e.g. microcephaly, craniostenosis.
d) Signs of raised intracranial pressure: in childhood, suture diastasis, copper-beaten appearance (less reliable): in adults, may be erosion of dorsum sellae.
e) Abnormal vascular channels, e.g. in vascular anomalies and some neoplasms.
f) Displacement of a calcified pineal gland.
g) Calcification of intracranial blood vessels, or calcification in some neoplasms.
h) Abnormalities of skull base and cervical spine alignment (may require special views) as in Arnold Chiari malformation.
i) Localised views or tomograms may show specific areas of abnormality, e.g. widening of internal auditory meatus with acoustic neuroma.

2. X-RAYS OF THE VERTEBRAL COLUMN may show:

a) Fractures.
b) Abnormal curvature.
c) Abnormal local or generalised bony structure, e.g. neoplasm, osteoporosis.
d) Abnormal shape of vertebrae, e.g. collapse, osteophyte formation.
e) Abnormal intervertebral spaces or foramina, encroachment by osteophytes, or tumours such as neurofibromas.
f) Abnormal intervertebral joints.
g) Calcification of extracranial vessels.
h) Abnormalities of spinal canal, e.g. widening due to neoplasm, narrowing due to prolapsed intervertebral disc.

3. LUMBAR PUNCTURE

Indications

Investigation of suspected:
a) Meningitis:
   (i) infective
   (ii) carcinomatous.
b) Subarachnoid haemorrhage.
c) Neurosyphilis (repeated 6 months and 2 years following treatment)

As part of myelographic investigation to look at:
a) Spinal cord and roots.
b) Disc spaces.
c) Cerebrospinal pathways for evidence of local block.

In treatment: injection of drugs for:
a) Tuberculous or other bacterial meningitis.
b) Leukaemic infiltration of the meninges.

Contraindications
a) Raised intracranial pressure.
b) Suspected space occupying lesion in the posterior fossa.
c) Suspected intracranial space occupying lesion above the tentorium.
d) Presence of ventricular dilatation and possible raised intracranial pressure.
e) Tissue suppuration near the puncture site.

4. CEREBROSPINAL FLUID CHANGES

	Normal range	Common abnormalities
Cells	less than 5 mm^3 (all lymphocytes)	Traumatic tap – blood clears in successive samples. Haemorrhage – uniformly blood-stained xanthochromia within 6 hours of a bleed, persists for three weeks. Cloudy fluid – if cells > 400/mm^3. Moderate increase in cells – trauma, recent air encephalogram, intracranial neoplasms. Marked increase in cells – bacterial (polymorphs) or viral (lymphocytes) meningitis, fungal infections.

Protein	15–45 mg% (infants up to 3 months normal limit up to 100 mg%)	a) *Increased up to several hundred mg%* *in* obstruction to C.S.F. pathways, may clot in tube (Froins' syndrome).
		b) *Albumino – cytologic dissociation* (*cells not increased markedly*) *may occur in:* C.S.F. obstruction and in Guillain-Barré syndrome.
		c) *Raised in:* Liver disorders, paraproteinaemias, chronic encephalitides, neurosyphilis, multiple sclerosis. Immunoglobulin G fraction raised in some patients with multiple sclerosis, and neurosyphilis.
Glucose	50–80 mg%	*Raised in:* diabetes mellitus. *Reduced in:* meningitis-carcinomatous (marked reduction), infective (marked reduction), tuberculous (moderate reduction), abscess (moderate or severe reduction-cell count dependent).

5. RETINAL EXAMINATION WITH FLUORESCEIN ANGIOGRAPHY

To ascertain presence of papilloedema when doubt exists.
Fluorescein leaks from capillaries into extravascular tissues in the presence of disc oedema, and stains the peripapillary retina for up to 10 minutes; none leaks when disc is normal.

6. COMPUTERISED AXIAL TOMOGRAPHY (CT SCAN)

Indicates:
a) Ventricular size and shape, e.g. hydrocephalus, cortical atrophy.
b) Pathological intracranial lesions (as small as 1 cm in diameter).
Reasonable assessment of:
a) Type of lesion, using tissue density measurements, e.g. infarction, haemorrhage, cystic lesions.
   Intravenous contrast injections can increase the definition of some lesions, e.g. neoplasm.
May miss:
a) Diffuse early lesions, e.g. microgliomatosis.
b) Very small localised lesions.
c) Small lesions in certain critical areas, e.g. near the base of the skull, near the anterior intracranial optic pathways.
d) Rarely — subdural haematoma if iso-dense with brain tissue on the scan.

7. ISOTOPE BRAIN SCAN

Technetium 99 m is the usual isotope.

May, but does not invariably, demonstrate intracranial neoplasms, e.g. meningiomas, vascular gliomas, metastases.

Poor indication of lesions in the posterior fossa.

8. MAGNETIC RESONANCE IMAGING (Relevant to the nervous system)

Advantages:
a) Painless, non-invasive.
b) Facility to image in several planes.
c) Absence of beam hardening artefact due to bone.
d) Availability of different sequences.
e) Absence of ionising radiation.
f) Better resolution of brainstem structures, spinal cord.
g) Can distinguish between cystic and solid lesions.
h) High degree of contrast between grey and white matter.
i) Shows up demyelinating plaques, cerebellar herniation, blood clot is well differentiated from the lumen of a blood vessel or an aneurysm.

Disadvantages:
a) Can still miss small intrinsic brain lesions, may fail to demonstrate small meningiomas.
b) Extent of oedema around a glioma or tumour may give rise to some difficulty in interpretation.
c) Calcification is not shown.
d) More time consuming than CT.
e) Special problems for patients on life support machines.
f) High capital and running costs.

Should be reserved for patients where diagnostic advantage well established.

9. ARTERIOGRAPHY

Mortality up to 0.25%.

Carotid, vertebral, or less commonly arch aortogram. Depending on vessel injected, will show intra and extracranial vessels, and presence or absence of:
a) Constriction of vessels.
b) Obstruction, e.g. by embolus.
c) Loss of vascular patterns, e.g. in arterial thrombosis.
d) Displacement, e.g. by space occupying lesions.

e) Pathological circulation in some neoplasms or vascular malformations.
f) Aneurysm formation.
g) Venous thrombosis.

10. X-RAY CONTRAST ENCEPHALOGRAPHY

Using air or myodil. Usually restricted to neurosurgical centres, and now performed after an initial CAT scan.

Neurophysiological investigations

1. ELECTROENCEPHALOGRAPHY (EEG)

Records electrical activity over the brain; usually over the scalp, rarely intracerebral.

a) *Electrodes*: usually 22, placed at uniform intervals, according to the International 10–20 system.

b) *Connections*: bipolar (2 electrodes) or monopolar to a specified reference electrode.

c) *Recording*: eyes open and closed, also 3 minutes hyperventilation, and brief photic stimulation at varying flicker rates.

d) *Activity*:
Delta: ½–3 Hz (cycles per second)
Theta: 4–7 Hz
Alpha: 8–13 Hz
Beta: 14–30 Hz

e) *Normal activity*: waking record — either alpha posteriorly (amplitude 25–100 μv), and beta anteriorly (amplitude approximately 15 μv), or generalised low amplitude beta.
Drowsiness — alpha intermittently decreased, theta appears.
Sleep — delta and some theta activity. Runs of fast activity — sleep spindles, and arousal 'K' complexes.
Children — varying amounts of slow activity, gradually replaced by alpha with increasing age.

f) *Abnormal activity*:
1. Reduced amount and amplitude of normal frequencies, and/or excess slow frequencies, can be generalised or localised.
2. Abnormal waveforms — sharp waves (transient waves of peaked outline, 70–200 msec duration); spikes (duration 20–70 msec); spike and slow wave complexes, either occurring spontaneously or in response to provocation by hyperventilation, photic stimulation or sleep.

NOTE: (i) A single normal EEG *never excludes* intracranial pathology, but in certain suspected conditions makes the diagnosis *very unlikely*, e.g. cerebral abscess, encephalitis, frequent apparent minor absences.

215

(ii) Serial recordings may show deterioration (e.g. with neoplasms) or improvement (e.g. after a cerebrovascular accident), therefore more helpful than a single record.

(iii) If generalised excess slow activity is seen, need to exclude metabolic causes, e.g. uraemia, electrolyte imbalance, hypoglycaemia, or liver failure before assuming primary intracerebral lesion.

g) *Indications for EEG*:
1. Differential diagnosis of episodic loss of consciousness.
2. Differentiation of focal attacks, e.g. temporal lobe epilepsy, focal motor or sensory symptomatic 'partial' epilepsy. Sleep recording can activate temporal lobe foci.
3. Serial assessments in epilepsy, e.g. may reveal developing neoplasm, or chronic degenerative condition. Useful in detailed preoperative assessment. If surgery, e.g. lobectomy, contemplated for intractable fits — bilateral foci a contraindication to surgery.
4. Serial examination helpful in distinguishing neoplasm from vascular lesion, may indicate a need to repeat CT scan.
5. Investigation of unexplained behaviour disorder in children can reveal undetected minor absences, temporal lobe foci, deteriorating cortical function, e.g. in cerebral degenerative disorders, or indicate possibility of brain damage at birth.
6. Investigation of suspected abscess, can indicate need for CT scan, e.g. in meningitis without focal signs.
7. Confirmation of brain death. Two *iso-electric* (flat) records, at intervals of 24 hours, using maximum amplification (10 μv/ cm). There must be no evidence of hypothermia or barbiturate intoxication, which are potentially reversible causes of a flat record. The Royal College's criteria do not require that an EEG is included for a diagnosis of brain death. If the criteria are not satisfied, that is the patient is still alive, an EEG may help to decide the degree of brain damage. The presence of electro-cerebral silence, in a patient who is not hypothermic or under the influence of drugs, is merely a sign of a very poor prognosis, rather than a sign that brain death has occurred.

h) *The EEG and epilepsy*: an EEG, *during* a major, focal, or minor fit, which shows specific ictal abnormality, *is diagnostic* of an epileptic attack. Conversely a generalised attack without appropriate simultaneous EEG changes indicates that that particular attack is not a genuine fit.

A normal interictal EEG does *not* exclude a diagnosis of epilepsy, which is primarily a clinical assessment based on the history and an eye witness account.

An abnormal interictal EEG may, but does not necessarily, indicate epilepsy. Generalised, episodic, interictal EEG spike and wave activity, with a history of attacks of loss of consciousness, gives support to a diagnosis of a liability to epilepsy.

Spike and wave EEG activity in response to photic stimulation, the photoconvulsive response — supports a diagnosis of a liability to fits, *but* also occurs in approximately 1% of normal children who never have fits. In psychomotor epilepsy and temporal lobe attacks, a routine and a sleep EEG will reveal spike foci in almost 90% of patients. *N.B.* Useful in assessing cause of episodic aggressive behaviour, but *rarely* of help in deciding if a criminal episode occurred during a fit.

Fit frequency and degree of EEG abnormality *not* closely related in major focal attacks, but definitely related in minor or petit mal attacks.

i) *Ambulatory EEG monitoring*: Combined EEG and ECG ambulatory recordings now invaluable for investigation of epileptic and other episodic attacks. Miniaturised amplifiers on the head, and a cassette tape recorder attached to the patient's waist allows recordings of seizure activity to continue over hours and days. The EEG and ECG activity is later replayed at modified speeds for analysis.

This form of monitoring can be combined with video recordings of clinical changes.

j) *Intensive care and prolonged EEG monitoring*: Changes in cerebral activity related to altered physiological conditions, or anaesthetic agents can be revealed by the EEG. The displayed activity usually needs to be condensed, and methods such as frequency or power spectral analysis are now incorporated in many commercial equipment items.

2. EVOKED POTENTIALS

a) Visually evoked potentials

Light stimulation causes an evoked response which can be recorded on the scalp over the occipital cortex. Averaging procedures improve the definition of the response. Stimulus may be a flashing light, but response is more uniform with alternating black and white checker board, which is reversed at a rate of 2 per second. The latency between stimulus and response, normally approximately 100 msec, is increased by damage to the optic nerve or intracranial visual pathways.

Optic neuritis causes significant delays in over 90% of patients. In patients with multiple sclerosis, both with and without known previous retrobulbar neuritis, the response is delayed in at least 70%.

b) Auditory evoked potentials
Scalp recordings of electrical responses to auditory stimuli always require averaging techniques for display, as amplitude only 0.5– 1 μv. Multiphasic responses have been identified and brain stem components delineated. In multiple sclerosis, brain stem components delayed in 46% of patients with appropriate signs, but delays also reported in over 50% of those without brain stem signs. *N.B.* Other pathological disturbance of brain stem function may also delay the responses.

c) Electrospinogram
Skin surface recordings over the cervical cord region, in response to electrical stimulation of the median nerve yield well defined potentials when averaging techniques employed. If delay in the peripheral nerve component is excluded, then any delay in latency reveals proximal abnormality. Increases have been reported in 64% of patients with multiple sclerosis without clinical signs to suggest cervical cord involvement.

d) Late cognitive potentials
Changes in brain electrical activity induced by alterations in behavioural patterns include the contingent negative variation (CNV), late as opposed to short latency or early evoked potentials, e.g. P300, and the Bereitschaftspotential. These are of use in the research laboratory to monitor sensitive psychological variables, but their clinical application and value is not yet generally accepted.

FURTHER READING

Binnie, C. D. (1983) Telemetric EEG monitoring in epilepsy. In *Recent Advances in Epilepsy*. ed Pedley, T. A. & Meldrum, B. S. pp. 155–178. Edinburgh: Churchill Livingstone.

Driver, M. V. & McGallivray, B. B. (1982) Electroencephalography. In *A Textbook of Epilepsy*. ed. Laidlaw, J. & Richens, A. pp. 155–195. Edinburgh: Churchill Livingstone.

Halliday, A. M., Butler, S. R. & Paul, R. (1987) *A Textbook of Clinical Neurophysiology*. Chichester: J. Wiley & Sons.

Jeavons, P. M. (1987) Photosensitive epilepsy. In *A Textbook of Epilepsy*. ed. Laidlaw, J. & Richens, A. pp. 195–226. Edinburgh: Churchill Livingstone.

Morgan, M. H. et al. (1987) The relative diagnostic values of visual evoked potentials (VEPs) and immunoglobulon estimations in multiple sclerosis. In *Multiple Sclerosis: Immunological, Diagnostic, and Therapeutic Aspects*. ed. Rose, F. C. & Jones, R. London: John Libbey.

Pedley, T. (1984) Epilepsy and the human EEG. In *Electrophysiology of Epilepsy*. ed. Schwartzkroin, P. A. & Wheal, H. V. pp 1–30. London: Academic Press.

5. SOME ABNORMAL EEGs

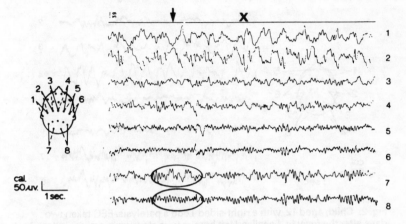

Fig. 1. Female patient, aged 40, with an extensive glioma in the left temporal lobe. The EEG shows localised slow waves over the left temporal area. In channels 1 and 2 there are delta waves and some show phase reversal, (↓) being deflected down in channel 1 and up in channel 2. Occasional single waves of sharp outline also show phase reversal between channels 1 and 2. (×) Alpha activity in channel 7 is less regular than in channel 8, and there are underlying theta and delta waves in channel 7 (◯).

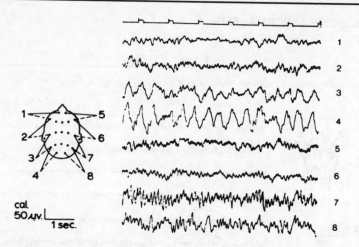

Fig. 2. Child, aged 12, with a right-sided Todd's paralysis. EEG taken two days after the focal fit. Localised left hemisphere slow wave activity is seen in channels 3 and 4. Subsequent investigations failed to reveal any obvious cause for the clinical manifestations. The child made a good recovery and the EEG returned to normal.

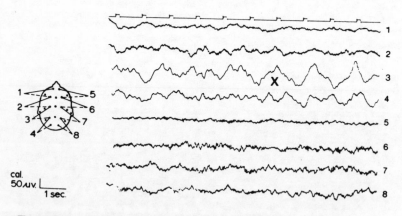

Fig. 3. Child, aged 8 months. Record shows unilateral delta waves (×) over the left hemisphere — especially in channels 3 and 4. This abnormality resulted from a prolonged right-sided fit in a child who had had infantile spasms at age 5 months, but whose CT scan was normal.

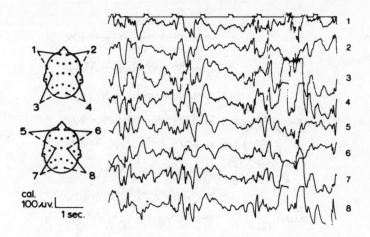

Fig. 4. Child, aged 5 months. Episodic bursts of high amplitude mixed spike and slow waves, separated by periodic suppression of electrical activity. Hypsarrhythmic EEG in a child with salaam spasms.

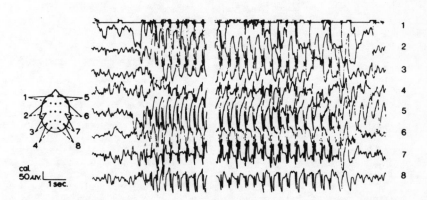

Fig. 5. Child, aged 7 years. Minor absences of petit mal type. EEG shows generalised spike and slow wave complexes starting and ceasing synchronously over all areas, during which the child failed to respond to simple commands.

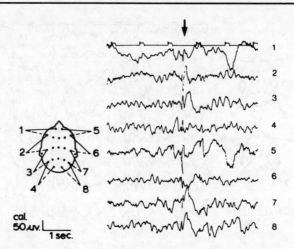

Fig. 6. 7-year-old child with grand mal epilepsy. Bilateral spike and slow wave discharges. Phase reversal of spike and slow wave components seen over both hemispheres, between channels 1 and 3, as well as 4 and 6. (↓)

PART THREE

On taking examinations

Examination technique and some common faults

This section discusses the errors which are commonly committed by both undergraduate and postgraduate candidates for examinations in psychiatry and suggests ways of avoiding them.

THE PAPERS

Multiple choice
It is important to attempt all the questions and a careful watch on the way you allocate your time is essential. It is never advisable to guess, because you can lose marks for wrong answers. Read the precise wording of each question carefully and allow time to go back over items on which you are not certain.

The essay paper
Again it is crucial that you budget your time efficiently. So often the amount written on successive questions becomes progressively smaller, and the bad candidate may furnish only a few scrappy lines as his last answer, sometimes with naive apologies. It is not possible to gain more than a limited number of marks for long answers but many can be lost through a failure to complete the paper adequately, and with a close marking system this is a most important point to remember.

A good essay answer should pay attention to the following points:

Legibility, coherence and style
Attention to basic English grammar and care over tidiness and legibility seem obvious points, but they are very frequently ignored. This of course implies a lack of consideration for the examiner, who is then in turn less inclined to give the borderline candidate any benefit of doubt.

Planning
An essay type answer should contain an introduction which sets out the general aims of the answer, a body and it should end with relevant conclusions. By all means use headings but avoid using

long and ill-explained lists. Do not waste time on pointless repetition and recapitulation.

Information

To omit important facts suggests carelessness or ignorance: errors of commission are clearly due to inadequate knowledge of the subject: irrelevance suggests lack of care in reading the question, poor judgement regarding what to include, or 'padding' because of inadequate command of the relevant facts.

The answer should cover all relevant aspects of the topic and it should avoid a too limited approach. For example, discussion of assessment should include special investigations as well as clinical evaluation and differential diagnosis: it may be necessary to refer to all age groups, though not uncommonly either children or adults are discussed as opposed to both.

An unduly restricted interpretation of the question is a very common fault. Another is the failure to include hard facts such as the absolute or relevant incidence of syndromes (for example that Alzheimer's Disease is far more common than Pick's Disease), the incidence of symptoms, or the proportion of patients responding to treatment. All these are relevant to clinical skills and judgement. A good postgraduate answer will also contain critical reference to the literature.

Explanation and definition

A poor candidate tends to indulge in the use of technical terms and concepts in a way which does not indicate whether he really understands them. It should be a golden rule that adequate explanation must be provided at all points and the answer should be liberally laced with phrases such as 'by which I mean', or 'by this is meant'. It is not sufficient to take technicalities for granted, assuming that the examiner understands them and that he will necessarily believe that you do too. Whenever a diagnostic entity such as depression is mentioned you should explain what you mean by it. All terms should be used with the utmost care: avoid those such as 'inadequate' or 'psychopathic' unless you are prepared to define them fully. These points are of course particularly important when new concepts such as 'high expressed emotion' or 'face to face contact' are being considered.

Critical and well-reasoned discussion

You should attempt to show that you can think for yourself as opposed to merely reproducing lists obtained from books, and that you can apply in a sensible way the concepts which you discuss in the light of adequate clinical experience and with a correct sense of priorities. Avoid a superficial approach and the use of clichés, for example by describing treatment merely as 'supportive psychotherapy involving a multidisciplinary approach with a social worker seeing the family and occupational therapy'. Each of these needs further explanation and justification. Unsatisfactory essay answers in clinical psychiatry, even in postgraduate examinations, are sometimes written at a level which could be produced by a well informed layman: the combination of superficiality of approach, failure to define technical terms which are used uncritically, all · contribute to a bad overall effect on the reader. Many of these errors are due to faulty examination technique and with adequate practice and preparation they can of course be avoided.

Reference to the clinical situation
In order to demonstrate that you can apply theoretical knowledge in practice, you should provide an essay answer which contains adequate reference to the relevant clinical situation. In this way theoretical issues can be explained more fully by illustrating how they may be applied.

You should also demonstrate that your priorities are correct and that you are able to distinguish between common and rare conditions, or hazardous from harmless procedures. You should try to show that you are sufficiently critical of the terms and concepts which you use by indicating the limitations of their application.

Breadth of approach
Although you may feel a certain partisan allegiance to one or more theoretical approach, you should do justice to all others which may be relevant: you must be able to show that you can evaluate a variety of viewpoints without prejudice. In discussing the causes or management of any condition make sure that you cover such aspects as epidemiological, social, psychological and nursing as well as more obvious clinical problems. Do not forget to consider differential diagnosis: few psychiatric syndromes are so well defined that no others are relevant, and take care to discuss all other possible contenders at all points. Do not deal with diagnostic categories as if they are disease entities akin to those of general medicine, but remember that most are loose descriptive syndromes: the best example of this error is the way reactive and endogenous depression are so often assumed to be mutually exclusive without any attempt being made to define the basis for distinguishing between the two.

Avoidance of other common errors
Do not make silly casual comments. If you bring in your personal experiences make sure that you do not base your answer entirely upon them: demonstrate that you also have an adequate knowledge of the literature and the views of others. If you mention authors only do so when you can furnish correct details of their findings otherwise you merely give the impression of 'name dropping'.
Avoid using your answer to indulge your views on irrelevant general

issues such as the state of society or other organisations and disciplines. Always ask yourself whether these matters are strictly relevant. Be precise over what you write, avoid unstructured verbosity and take care over how you express your ideas. The candidate who wrote 'criminal shop lifters should be eliminated' produced a rather comic effect which was probably unintended but which did nothing to add to the quality of his answer.

THE CLINICAL M.R.C.Psych. EXAMINATION
(Membership exam: see later for the new Part I examination)

The precise form will of course vary according to the particular examination being taken. The M.R.C.Psych. examination allows the candidate one hour to assess his patient (for details of Part I see later) and this is followed by a five minute review period during which he gathers his ideas together before being interviewed by two examiners for a total of 30 minutes on matters relevant to his case.

In this examination the 'clinical' is regarded as a crucial part of the test and must be passed. Adequate attention to examination strategy is nowhere more important than here.

Patient assessment
In order to work as quickly as possible, a systematic approach to the history and mental state is essential. You will be expected to carry out a physical examination (usually restricted in extent) if you think it is relevant to the particular problem with which you are dealing. In any case it is probably advisable to allow the last few minutes or so to check the blood pressure, optic fundi and reflexes, if only rather summarily: sometimes something unexpected and surprising turns up and you will then be likely to earn extra marks. Remember that you can still carry on talking to your patient whilst checking physical signs and so elaborate on gaps in the history if necessary.

The review period
During this time you must assemble the relevant positive points clearly in your mind. A good way of doing this is to prepare a summary from the notes which you have made during your interview with the patient. In the M.R.C.Psych. examination it is assumed that candidates will have organised their findings and conclusions in this way before they proceed to interview with the examiners. The candidate's task is not made easier by the fact that the term 'formulation' can have a variety of meanings and as a result its use is discouraged. The following scheme has the advantage that it promotes a comprehensive summary of all the available data. Such an approach is essential in the face of a bewildering variety of information. It forces you to commit yourself with regards to what is relevant and to a logical systematic approach. It should also give you confidence because its systematic approach helps you to remember the relevant facts. The candidate

who proceeds to meet the examiner without having to search nervously through a mass of notes and one who can speak from memory creates a good impression immediately. Practice at presentation permits this to be done.

An adequate case presentation has the following headings:

Descriptive: a few sentences summarising the essence of the history and mental state. This should take two or three minutes only.

Diagnostic: your first choice syndrome and you will need to justify it.

Differential diagnostic: the other possibilities with points for and against.

Aetiological: include all types of possible causes.

Psychodynamic: outline any themes which are discernible.

Therapeutic: how you would proceed in management.

Prognostic: what you think the likely outcome will be.

You should take care to consider these aspects of the clinical problem in the above logical sequence because failure to do so leads to confusion. Never consider treatment before summarising the clinical features and diagnosis. The new M.R.C. Psych. examination Part I clinical will be concerned with assessment, investigation and diagnosis, but *not* with management (see later).

Interview with examiners

To have a systematic and comprehensive method of presentation allows you confidence when you proceed to your interview with the examiners. At some point you may be asked to re-interview your patient very briefly in the presence of the examiners in order to illustrate the main symptoms of mental phenomenon. Your relationship with your patient, your ability to put him at ease and your skill with which you handle a brief yet relevant discussion will be evaluated at this point.

You can anticipate some predictable opening gambits on the part of the examiner who may say 'tell me about your patient' or 'what is your diagnosis'. Some candidates react by starting on a long detailed discussion of the case history which includes many irrelevancies, and after 5–10 minutes have to be stopped by the examiner. Such a false start situation is harmful: it puts you off your stride and wastes time in which valuable marks might otherwise have been gained. It is best to anticipate and avoid this kind of difficulty by being explicit about your approach and to warn the examiner in advance how you would like to answer his initial question. For example it might be appropriate in response to 'tell me about your patient' to say 'I would like to answer that by summarising very briefly the main positive findings on assessment and then proceed under the headings diagnosis, differential diagnosis, aetiology, psychopathology, therapy and prognosis.'

Many candidates are so anxious that they become over-inclusive: they are afraid to summarise their findings and opinions and are reluctant to opt for diagnostic priorities. They clutch their notes nervously and scan the examiner's face for inspiration. You will appear far more confident if you are armed with a systematic approach which allows you to summarise the facts and to present the case in a fluent and logical way. So often the examiner is faced with an immensely detailed yet haphazard account and he has to interrupt repeatedly in a search for relevant data. The candidate who can proceed logically through a seven point formulation which has been suggested here cannot fail to impress.

Be prepared for interruptions and don't be put off by them: practice being interviewed by your fellow trainees in this way. Argue your point firmly and try not to shift your ground just to please the examiner or to sound out his views before starting to state yours. If you don't know, say so and do not hedge.

Do not look for hidden traps and try to avoid an argument. Remember that the examiner who seems unduly critical may well appear so because he thinks you are doing well and so he is trying to find out the full extent of your knowledge by asking difficult and exacting questions. Control your own emotional reaction to what happens in the interview and try to deal with each point systematically rather than in a haphazard way. As in essay writing, try to define all the terms you use and do not use them loosely.

THE M.R.C. Psych. ORALS

These usually consist of a series of questions covering a wide range of topics which may or may not be relevant to any speciality in which you work. Try to provide crisp relevant answers. Questions may be asked during a 30 minute period on any aspect of psychiatric disorders and their management. In the M.R.C. Psych. examination the focus is entirely upon clinical assessment and management (see later). Remember that the examiner will want to pass the candidate who has adequate knowledge, who can evaluate it critically, and who demonstrates that he has had clinical experience sufficient to apply it with a good sense of priority and judgement.

In preparing for examinations candidates far too often invest an excessive amount of their time in learning a very great deal of small print material from text books. It would be far better if more time could be spent in practising case presentation and discussion of basic topics with colleagues or tutors. This of course needs more planning and organisation in one's learning and revision, compared with comfortable arm-chair reading. Such an approach is well worth the effort, however, and will help you to avoid many basic errors which frequently contribute to failure in clinical examinations.

THE NEW M.R.C. Psych. EXAMINATION AND ITS IMPLICATIONS

The examination for Membership of the Royal College of Psychiatrists, which began in 1971, is currently undergoing a major reorganisation.

In its previous form, the examination was divided into two parts: the Preliminary Test, concerned mainly with sciences basic to psychiatry, was followed some three years later by the Membership Examination itself. Several aspects of this approach have been the subject of criticism, the most consistent being the absence of any clinical test during the first three years of training, the implicit encouragement to disregard the study of basic sciences after passing the Preliminary Test, the limited reliability of marking the essay paper, and poor integration of the examination with the educational process as a whole. The several changes inherent in the new examination aim to remedy these acknowledged deficiencies.

The previous style examination will continue until 1992 in order to allow those who have passed its preliminary test to complete the whole examination.

THE GENERAL AIM OF THE NEW EXAMINATION

The examination will still serve as the criterion of successful general postgraduate professional training. This should be completed before proceeding to a period of Higher Training which then prepares the trainee for the autonomous responsibilities of being a consultant. The examination will continue to consist of two parts and the emphasis will still focus on general psychiatry, with the inclusion of specialty expertise at an appropriate level.

The new Part 1 examination

The new arrangements represent a major shift of emphasis. The Part 1 is to become an examination in basic clinical psychiatry, testing this plus certain relevant aspects of basic sciences and practical skills equivalent to one year of training. It will in effect have greater relevance than the previous preliminary test to what the trainee actually does during the first year, and will consist of a multiple choice paper and a clinical examination.

These changes constitute a major challenge to both candidates and examiners. The MCQ paper will be concerned with basic psychopathology — descriptive and explanatory, clinical assessment, diagnosis, clinical pharmacology and the neurosciences. The examiners will need to be very clear about exactly how much detail should be required at this stage of training and to work out ways of assessing basic knowledge whilst allowing for limits in detailed theoretical understanding.

The Part 1 clinical is perhaps the most challenging innovation of all. It will aim to test basic clinical skills, including history taking, and evaluating the mental state (as well as assessment of key physical signs where relevant, although a physical examination will not routinely be expected), followed by a succinct, accurate outline of diagnosis and assessment. In the Part 1 clinical management will not be included. The examiners will want to evaluate basic clinical skills, what is asked, how it is asked and the manner in which the candidate relates to the patient.

In the Part 1 clinical examination a *good clinical history* will be:
— systematic
— comprehensive
— coherent and internally consistent
— relevant and will avoid unnecessary detail
— multidimensional in approach (physical, psychological, social)
— accurate
— able to distinguish fact/opinion, description/explanation, direct/indirect data.

In the Part 1 clinical examination a *good clinical interview technique* will:
— be flexible (form and content)
— be goal directed (but not a checklist approach)
— be sensitive and controlled (but not interrogational)
— allow the patient to talk
— use open rather than leading questions
— include summary statements and clarifications.

In the Part 1 clinical examination *the candidate should aim to demonstrate*:
— tact and consideration for the patient
— sensitivity to the patient's problems and mental state
— empathy
— control of the interview
— self control (tolerant of frustration, ambiguity, uncertainties)
— objectivity (avoid partisan attitude towards one theoretical approach).

The new Part 2 examination
This will be an examination in the sciences basic to psychiatry and in clinical topics covering general psychiatry and the subspecialties. The trainee will therefore need to be prepared on a much wider front than previously, and the examination will be concerned particularly with the integration between basic sciences and clinical issues.
There will be five parts: an essay paper (one essay only), MCQ (basic sciences), short answer question paper, a second MCQ paper (clinical topics), the clinical examination and a patient management problem oral. A pass in the clinical will be mandatory, and all but one of the others must be passed at one time, the pass mark being a 50% aggregate.

The trainee who is anxious about exactly how much detailed knowledge of basic sciences will be expected should find reassurance in the fact that basic knowledge, general principles,